MELATONIN
in the
PROMOTION
of HEALTH

CRC SERIES IN MODERN NUTRITION
Edited by Ira Wolinsky and James F. Hickson, Jr.

Published Titles

Manganese in Health and Disease, Dorothy J. Klimis-Tavantzis
Nutrition and AIDS: Effects and Treatments, Ronald R. Watson
Nutrition Care for HIV-Positive Persons: A Manual for Individuals and Their Caregivers,
    Saroj M. Bahl and James F. Hickson, Jr.
Calcium and Phosphorus in Health and Disease, John J.B. Anderson and
    Sanford C. Garner

Edited by Ira Wolinsky

Published Titles

Handbook of Nutrition in the Aged, Ronald R. Watson
Practical Handbook of Nutrition in Clinical Practice, Donald F. Kirby and
    Stanley J. Dudrick
Handbook of Dairy Foods and Nutrition, Gregory D. Miller, Judith K. Jarvis, and
    Lois D. McBean
Advanced Nutrition: Macronutrients, Carolyn D. Berdanier
Childhood Nutrition, Fima Lifschitz
Antioxidants and Disease Prevention, Harinda S. Garewal
Nutrition and Cancer Prevention, Ronald R. Watson and Siraj I. Mufti
Nutrition and Health: Topics and Controversies, Felix Bronner
Nutritional Concerns of Women, Ira Wolinsky and Dorothy J. Klimis-Tavantzis
Nutrients and Gene Expression: Clinical Aspects, Carolyn D. Berdanier
Advanced Nutrition: Micronutrients, Carolyn D. Berdanier
Nutrition and Women's Cancers, Barbara Pence and Dale M. Dunn
Nutrients and Foods in AIDS, Ronald R. Watson
Melatonin in the Promotion of Health, Ronald R. Watson

Forthcoming Titles

Advanced Human Nutrition, Denis Medeiros and Robert E.C. Wildman
Child Nutrition in Developing Countries, Noel W. Solomons
Concepts in Fitness Programming, Robert G. McMurray
Handbook of Nutrition for Vegetarians, Joan Sabaté and Rosemary A. Ratzin
Laboratory Tests for the Assessment of Nutritional Status, Second Edition, H.E.
    Sauberlich
Management of Stress and Eating Disorders for Women and Children, Jacalyn J. Robert
Nutrition and the Eye, Allen Taylor
Nutrition in Space Flight and Weightlessness Models, Helen W. Lane and
    Dale A. Schoeller
Nutrition: Chemistry and Biology, Second Edition, Julian H. Spallholz,
    L. Mallory Boylan, and Judy A. Driskell
Nutritional Anemias, Usha Ramakrishnan
Tryptophan: Biochemicals and Health Implications, Herschel Sidransky

MELATONIN
in the
PROMOTION
of HEALTH

Edited by

RONALD R. WATSON, Ph.D.

CRC Press
Boca Raton   London   New York   Washington, D.C.

Library of Congress Cataloging-in-Publication Data

Melatonin in the promotion of health / edited by Ronald R. Watson
      p.   cm. — (Modern nutrition)
      Includes bibliographical references and index.
      ISBN 0-8493-8564-4
      1. Melatonin—Physiological effect.   2. Melatonin—Health aspects.
I. Watson, Ronald R. (Ronald Ross)   II. Series: Modern nutrition
(Boca Raton, Fla.)
      [DNLM: 1. Melatonin—physiology. 2. Melatonin—therapeutic use.
WK 102 M517 1998]
QP572.M44M46   1998
612.4'92—dc21
DNLM/DLC
For Library of Congress   98-45986
                                                                CIP

Series Preface for Modern Nutrition

The CRC Series in Modern Nutrition is dedicated to providing the widest possible coverage of topics in nutrition. Nutrition is an interdisciplinary, interprofessional field par excellence. It is noted by its broad range and diversity. We trust the titles and authorship in this series will reflect that range and diversity.

Published for a broad audience, the volumes in the CRC Series in Modern Nutrition are designed to explain, review, and explore present knowledge and recent trends, developments, and advances in nutrition. As such, they will appeal to professionals as well as to the educated layman. The format for the series will vary with the needs of the author and the topic, including, but not limited to, edited volumes, monographs, handbooks, and texts.

Contributors from any bona fide area of nutrition, including the controversial, are welcome, just as I welcome the timely contribution of the book, *Melatonin in the Promotion of Health,* edited by my productive colleague, Ronald R. Watson.

Ira Wolinsky, Ph.D.
University of Houston
Series Editor

Preface

Melatonin is a hormone with well-recognized activities and the potential to influence many bodily functions. A derivative of tryptophan, melatonin is a powerful antioxidant with numerous effects on the metabolism, nutritional status, and health in the aging. It is being studied extensively as a key to understanding many of the nutritional and metabolic changes associated with diseases of aging. Supplementation with melatonin in humans and various model systems are testing theories of aging, as well as the role of oxidants and antioxidants in its disease processes. Restoration of melatonin production lost with increasing age has been shown to modify the actions of aging on lipid production, lipid peroxidation, tissue antioxidants, and cell functions. In addition to regulating certain aspects of aging, melatonin plays important roles in AIDS and some cancers by modulating metabolism and antioxidant nutrient status. Therefore, it is very timely to understand the role of the antioxidant melatonin, which is found in foods and is now being used extensively by the general public as a nonprescription nutritional supplement.

The primary focus of this book is to have experts review the potential effects of a loss of pineal function and the subsequent reduction in melatonin production, as well as its replacement as therapy. Therefore, the role of melatonin in Alzheimer's disease, reproduction, cancer, neurological functions, kidney activity, changes in body fat, and antioxidant activities are reviewed in depth. A variety of peptides are synthesized by the pineal gland, in addition to melatonin. While melatonin is the most extensively studied, other peptides also show biological activity; therefore, two chapters are devoted to neuropeptides from the pineal gland, their structure, and functions. Finally, the mechanisms of action including binding sites and non-pineal production are summarized.

About the Editor

Ronald R. Watson, Ph.D., initiated and directed the Specialized Alcohol Research Center at the University of Arizona College of Medicine until 1994. A theme of the facility's National Institute of Alcohol Abuse and Alcoholism (NIAAA) Center grant has been to understand the role of immunosuppression in murine AIDS, including the use of nutrition to normalize immune dysfunction. This has led to the use of antioxidants to treat immune dysfunction in mice due to age and/or murine AIDS. Dr. Watson currently directs an NIH grant and a study of oxidation and its immune enhancement of cardiotoxicity in murine AIDS. He is also funded to study the effects of melatonin on the elderly human.

Dr. Watson attended the University of Idaho and graduated from Brigham Young University in Provo, UT, with a degree in chemistry in 1966. He completed his Ph.D. degree in biochemistry in 1971 at Michigan State University. His postdoctoral schooling was completed at the Harvard School of Public Health in nutrition and microbiology, including two years of postdoctoral research in immunology. He was Assistant Professor of Immunology and conducted research at the University of Mississippi Medical Center in Jackson from 1973 to 1974. He was an Assistant Professor of Microbiology and Immunology at Indiana University Medical School from 1974 to 1978, and an Associate Professor at Purdue University in the Department of Food and Nutrition from 1978 to 1982. In 1982, he joined the faculty of the University of Arizona in the Department of Family and Community Medicine, Nutrition Section, and is a Research Professor in the Arizona Prevention Center. He has published 450 research papers and review chapters and edited 42 books.

Dr. Watson is a member of several national and international nutrition, immunology, and AIDS research societies. He directed the first symposium on nutrition and AIDS at FASEB and also at the International Congress on Nutrition in Australia in 1993. In 1997, he addressed the International Congress on Nutrition in Montreal on the subject of hormones and AIDS.

The Contributors

Rolf G.G. Anderson, Ph.D.
Department of Medicine and Care
Division of Pharmacology
Faculty of Health Sciences
Linköping, Sweden

Timothy J. Bartness, Ph.D.
Department of Psychology, and
Department of Biology,
   Neuropsychology, and Behavioral
   Neuroscience
Georgia State University
Atlanta, Georgia

Bryant Benson, Ph.D.
Department of Cell Biology
   and Anatomy
College of Medicine
University of Arizona
Tucson, Arizona

Gregory M. Brown, Ph.D.
Clarke Institute of Psychiatry
Toronto, Ontario, Canada

George A. Bubenik, M.D.
Department of Zoology
University of Guelph
Guelph, Ontario, Canada

William T. Cummings, Ph.D.
Arizona Prevention Center
University of Arizona
Tucson, Arizona

Jacqueline B. Fine, Ph.D.
Department of Medicine
Division of Geriatrics
Emory University School of Medicine
Atlanta, Georgia

John C. George, Ph.D.
Department of Zoology
University of Guelph
Guelph, Ontario, Canada

Paula Inserra, Ph.D.
Arizona Prevention Center
University of Arizona
Tucson, Arizona

Alexander Ivanovich Kuzmenko, Ph.D.
A.V. Palladin Institute of Biochemistry
Ukrainian National Academy
   of Sciences
Kiev, Ukraine

Bailin Liang, Ph.D.
Arizona Prevention Center
University of Arizona
Tucson, Arizona

Paolo Lissoni, Ph.D.
Division of Radiotherapy and Oncology
San Gerardo Hospital
Monza, Italy

Lena G.E. Mårtensson, Ph.D.
Department of Medicine and Care
Division of Pharmacology
Faculty of Health Sciences
Linköping, Sweden

Charles P. Maurizi, M.D.
Department of Pathology
Houston Medical Center
Warner Robins, Georgia

Rein Pähkla, Ph.D.
Department of Pharmacology
University of Tartu
Tartu, Estonia

Shiu-Fun Pang, Ph.D.
Department of Physiology
University of Hong Kong
Hong Kong, China

Lembit Rägo, Ph.D.
Department of Pharmacology
University of Tartu
Tartu, Estonia

Melvin Silverman, Ph.D.
MRC Membrane Biology Group
Department of Medicine
University of Toronto
Toronto, Ontario, Canada

David Solkoff, B.S.
Arizona Prevention Center
University of Arizona
Tucson, Arizona

Yong Song, Ph.D.
MRC Membrane Biology Group
Department of Medicine
University of Toronto
Toronto, Ontario, Canada

Ronald R. Watson, Ph.D.
Arizona Prevention Center
University of Arizona
Tucson, Arizona

Contents

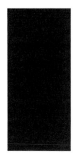

Chapter

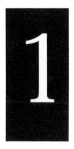

Melatonin Binding Sites

Lena G.E. Mårtensson and Rolf G.G. Andersson

Contents

Introduction

Melatonin binding sites are being investigated with increasing intensity, and knowledge in this area has accumulated rapidly since the development of radioligand binding assays for melatonin and the cloning of the ML-1 receptor. Today, there is somewhat of a consensus concerning both the structure and the pharmacological profile of the ML-1 receptor,[1] but there is no direct evidence of just what physiological role this receptor plays in most tissues. An interesting debate is in progress regarding all of the other melatonin binding sites. The putative ML-2 receptor, which has higher affinity for *N*-acetyl-serotonin than for melatonin, has not yet been cloned, and so far it has been detected only in binding studies on hamster and mouse.[2,3] What appear to be melatonin binding sites have also been found in cytoplasmic fractions.[4] Those sites may represent the intracellular receptors RZRα (cloned from human umbilical endothelial cells) and RZRβ (cloned from rat brain), which were originally detected as orphan receptors, and they may interact with melatonin in order to modulate inflammatory responses.[5] Moreover, we[6] used a bioassay based on fish melanophores and found evidence that melatonin interacts with the adrenergic system by modulating the α_2-adrenoceptor in an unknown way. Melatonin may also modulate several intracellular regulating processes by binding and inhibiting calmodulin.[7] The relevance of binding sites other than the ML-1 receptor is not known but is definitely of interest.

In this review we focus primarily on pharmacological aspects of the melatonin binding sites and discuss melatonin pharmacology in the perspective of possible receptors and physiological responses.

Methods

Binding Studies

Most of the reports of melatonin binding sites are based on results obtained with autoradiography or membrane binding assays (for methodological reviews, see References 8 to 10). Autoradiography is performed on thin tissue sections that have been incubated with different amounts of [^{125}I]melatonin and subsequently placed on an X-ray film. After development of the film, black areas suggest the presence of melatonin binding sites. To exclude unspecific binding sites (i.e., nonreceptor sites), experiments are carried out with [^{125}I]melatonin in combination with abundant amounts of nonradioactive melatonin, and the difference between the radioactive and nonradioactive forms represents the specific binding. By using different concentrations of [^{125}I]melatonin, it is possible to calculate the equilibrium dissociation constant (K_d) and the maximal binding (B_{max}) of the specific melatonin binding sites to be studied.

Radioligand experiments can also be performed on different cellular fractions. To study membrane binding, tissue is first homogenized and centrifuged at high speed to obtain a plasma membrane fraction containing possible melatonin binding sites. Thereafter, incubation with radioactive [^{125}I]melatonin, in the presence or absence of nonradioactive melatonin, is carried out in the same way as for autoradiography. After incubation, the samples are filtered through glass-fiber filters, and the amount of radiolabeled melatonin on the filter is measured in a gamma counter, and affinity and receptor density are calculated. Moreover, by using nonradioactive displacement substances other than melatonin, and comparing their efficacy in

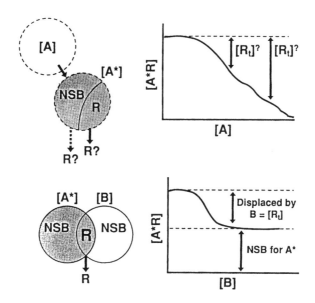

FIGURE 1
Definition of specific binding of a radioactive ligand [A*] by excess nonradioactive [A] may define nonreceptor sites as receptors. Definition of specific binding by a chemically nonrelated receptor ligand may eliminate problems with [A*] binding to nonreceptor sites. (From Kenakin, T., *Pharmacological Analysis of Drug-Receptor Interaction,* Raven Press, New York, 1993, p. 389. With permission.)

displacing [^{125}I]melatonin from its binding sites, a pharmacological profile can be proposed for the melatonin binding sites.

There are some methodological problems that should be considered. In general, iodonated melatonin is used because of the low density of the melatonin receptors in many preparations; this requires a ligand with high specific activity and, in most systems, is the only possibility for detecting binding at all. On the other hand, Kennaway and coworkers[10] have shown that the kinetics of iodonated melatonin is slower and not fully displaced by the unlabeled ligand. When using iodonated melatonin, not all of the measured binding can be inhibited by unlabeled melatonin, whereas the use of tritiated melatonin results in rapid and complete inhibition of the radioligand by the unlabeled ligand.

Very large amounts of unlabeled substances, usually melatonin, are also used in binding experiments. This can be somewhat troublesome, because large amounts of unlabeled melatonin may well compete for melatonin binding sites that, although specific, are actually non-receptor sites (i.e., proteins in the tissue preparation that can bind the radioligand in the same way receptor proteins do).[11-13] Such a situation would entail further disadvantages, as most studies use unlabeled ligands that are chemically similar to iodomelatonin (e.g., melatonin, *N*-acetyl-serotonin, and iodomelatonin itself). The similarity of the radioligand and the unlabeled ligand may increase the probability that melatonin will bind to non-receptor binding sites (Figure 1).[13]

Expression Studies

Cloning of the melatonin receptor has made it possible to transfect certain cell lines with cDNA for the melatonin receptor and thereby effect expression of melatonin receptors on the plasma membranes of the experimental cells.[14,15] Such methodology diminishes the problem of low melatonin receptor density and actually leads to overexpression (i.e., receptor density is increased to an above-normal level). This type of receptor-overexpressed system will probably promote ligand-receptor affinity, and it may also represent a suitable model for investigating G-protein interaction as a means of elucidating signal transduction pathways. Nevertheless, there may be pharmacological differences that make it difficult to translate the result of receptor-overexpression studies into an *in vivo* or an *in vitro* situation.[16]

In Vitro Systems

Nearly all of the sites that have been found to bind melatonin in binding assays are subject to speculation because they lack a corresponding physiological response, perhaps due to low site density or because most of the sites are located within the central nervous system (CNS). Only a few *in vitro* systems have been found to be affected by melatonin. By far the most well-known and experimentally most successful system comprises the chromatophores known as melanophores, which contain dispersible black pigment granules. Indeed, melatonin was discovered and named because of its ability to condense pigment granules in the center of amphibian melanophores.[17] Since that time, a method of culturing melanophores has been developed, and the ML-1 receptor has been cloned from an immortalized melanophore cell line.[14] Another very important *in vitro* system involves melatonin-induced inhibition of dopamine release in retina.[18] Moreover, other systems used *in vitro* take advantage of several additional effects exerted by melatonin, such as the fact that the hormone induces vascular contraction in rat caudal artery,[19] modulates secretion in human platelets,[20,21] increases human myometrial activity,[22] and inhibits cell growth in some cultured cells.[23,24]

Pharmacological Profile and Distribution of the ML-1 Receptor

The ML-1 receptor (Figure 2) was cloned in 1994.[14] It shows major similarities with known melatonin binding sites, and the receptor is a member of the seven-transmembrane receptor superfamily and is coupled to G-proteins. It has been suggested that signal transduction for the ML-1 receptor entails a cAMP decrease that is mediated by a pertussis-sensitive G_i-protein,[14,25] although other signal transduction pathways may be involved as well.[26,27] The pharmacological profile of the receptor has been elucidated in both pharmacological and radioligand binding studies, implying the

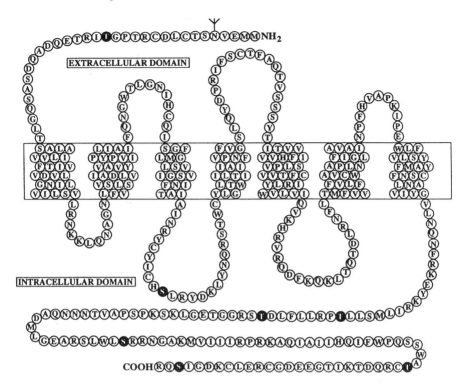

FIGURE 2

Proposed membrane structure of the *Xenopus* melatonin receptor. Deduced amino acid sequence is shown. Ψ = potential *N*-linked glycosylation site; solid circles = consensus sites for protein kinase C phosphorylation. (From Ebisawa, T., Karne, S., Lerner, M.R., and Reppert, S.M., *Proc. Natl. Acad. Sci. USA*, 91, 6135, 1994. With permission.)

following order of potency: I-melatonin > melatonin >> *N*-acetyl-serotonin. The K_d for melatonin is in the low picomolar range for the high-affinity state and in the higher picomolar range for the low-affinity state. Cloning experiments performed after the initial cloning of the receptor have shown that the ML-1 receptor family comprises three subtypes, designated ML-1a, b, and c (Table 1).[28] In all of the species studied, including humans, the ML-1a receptor is most abundant in the CNS, and the ML-1b is probably most abundant in retina.[29] ML-1c has been detected in *Xenopus* melanophores and in chickens and zebra fish, and, at least in chicken, ML-1a and ML-1c mRNA show varying distribution in the brain.[30] In general, the pharmacological profiles of the three subtypes are similar.

In the Central Nervous System

The ML-1 receptor has been studied primarily by use of autoradiographic assays of the CNS, and the results show large differences among species. At least in mammals,

TABLE 1
Characteristics of the Cloned G
Protein-Coupled Melatonin Receptors

Characteristic	Melatonin Receptor Subtypes		
	ML-1a	ML-1b	ML-1c
Clones:			
Human	Yes	Yes	No
Chicken	Yes	Yes[a]	Yes
Xenopus	Yes[a]	Yes[a]	Yes
Zebrafish	Yes[a]	Yes[a,b]	Yes[a]
K_d $(pM)^c$	20–40	160	20–60
Inhibition cAMP	Yes	Yes	Yes
Potency	2IMEL	2IMEL	2IMEL
	> MEL	> MEL	> MEL
	≥ 6CIMEL	= 6CIMEL	≥ 6CIMEL
	> NA5-HT	> NA5-HT	> NA5-HT
	>> 5-HT	>> 5-HT	>> 5-HT

[a] Fragment cloned; full-length coding region not cloned and expressed.

[b] Two fragments isolated, both falling in Mel-1a group by bootstrap analysis.

[c] K_d determined using 2-[^{125}I]iodomelatonin. 2IMEL = 2-iodomelatonin; MEL = melatonin; 6CIMEL = 6-chloromelatonin; NA5-HT = N-acetyl-5-hydroxytryptamine.

Source: From Reppert, S.M., Weaver, D.R., and Godson, C., *Trends Pharmacol. Sci.,* 17, 101, 1996. With permission.

the areas of greatest receptor density are found in the suprachiasmatic nucleus (SCN) in the hypothalamus, which is believed to be the center for the endogenous clock, and in the pars tuberalis of the pituitary, which probably regulates seasonal breeding. Other locations are also possible and may be dependent on sex, age, or species.

The melatonin binding sites in pars tuberalis have been studied in several seasonal breeders (for references, see Reference 31). A correlation between melatonin receptor density in pars tuberalis and the gonadal status has been noted. Short photoperiods induce a reduction in receptor density and a corresponding gonadal regression in Syrian hamsters,[32] and in the hedgehog the melatonin receptor density is much lower in autumn when the animals are sexually inactive.[33] It may be possible that lower melatonin receptor densities within the pars tuberalis are associated with sexually inactive animals in long-day breeders. The more precise mechanisms behind this hypothalamic-pituitary-gonadal axis are not known, although melatonin may regulate the GnRH generator and inhibit the short loop of luteinizing hormone (LH) and thereby inhibit ovulation and testosterone production.[34,35] Circulating testosterone levels in European hamsters have no effect on the density of melatonin receptors in pars tuberalis, which strengthens the possibility that pars tuberalis mediates the melatonin message into seasonal reproduction behavior.[32]

There is also some evidence of seasonality in regard to human fertility.[36–38] For those who live in the northern part of Europe, it has always been evident that more babies are born in springtime, and it has been confirmed that the rate of conception is higher during summer. Nevertheless, the presence of melatonin binding sites in the pars tuberalis is not as evident in humans as in other mammalian species. In postmortem materials, melatonin binding sites were not found throughout the pars tuberalis,[39] but the number of investigated tissue samples in that study was low and only one of the samples originated from a spontaneously cycling woman. Although human seasonal fertility may be due to causes other than decreasing melatonin secretion during summer, it is possible that melatonin is involved in some other way instead.

The density of melatonin binding sites is greater in the CNS of birds than in that of mammals. Binding data suggest only one receptor site in birds, but, in cloning experiments on the chicken,[30] two receptor subtypes were found — species homologues of ML-1a and ML-1c — which may reflect a subtype-selective distribution. In contrast to mammals, birds have no discrete melatonin binding site associated with the pars tuberalis. Instead, they have high-affinity melatonin binding sites within the visual system which may serve to modulate functions associated with sight, as many aspects of avian behavior (e.g., singing) vary with the time of day. Melatonin binding sites have been found within the song control systems of zebra finch and the canary.[40]

Interestingly, melatonin binding sites have been detected in a species of fish which lives in the deep sea, where it is impossible to rely on light for seasonal cycling.[41] The melatonin binding sites of this species (which have the pharmacological profile of an ML-1 receptor) are not distributed in the optical areas or in the cerebellum, as in many other animals including shallow waters fishes, but instead are located in the midbrain tegmentum and in the hindbrain. This suggests that the seasonal cycles are induced by stimuli other than light, perhaps through chemo- or mechanoreception, but that melatonin still may be involved.

The supposed endogenous clock — the suprachiasmatic nucleus — stimulates the circadian pineal synthesis of melatonin. SCN is inhibited by light, and during darkness the SCN sends impulses to the pineal gland that induce synthesis and secretion of melatonin.[42] Considering that, it is not surprising that the SCN is one of the areas with the largest populations of melatonin receptors. The exact cellular mechanisms of the SCN melatonin receptors have not been revealed, but they probably involve coordination of the endogenous clock and melatonin secretion. The melatonin receptor found in the SCN was the first human melatonin receptor to be cloned, and it was later subtyped as an ML-1a receptor.[43,44]

The melatonin binding properties in the SCN exhibit a circadian rhythm, and this may be due to the amount of circulating melatonin, as in the pars tuberalis. However, in an investigation of melatonin receptor density in rat SCN, pinealectomized rats displayed the same rhythm as control animals, suggesting that melatonin receptors are not regulated by circulating melatonin levels.[45] On the other hand, if the rats were kept in constant light or darkness, the rhythm disappeared. This implies that melatonin receptor density in the SCN and in the pars tuberalis are regulated by two different mechanisms, perhaps because these two areas perform different function.

In Retina

Melatonin receptors have been found in both mammalian and avian retina. A breakthrough in melatonin research occurred in the 1980s, when Dubocovic[18,46] studied rabbit retina and was the first to demonstrate functional melatonin receptors in mammalian neural tissue. Ducovich found that picomolar concentrations of melatonin could potently inhibit dopamine release in the rabbit retina, and suggested that this action is probably mediated through calcium-dependent inhibition of the release via a presynaptic receptor. This *in vitro* system is important in melatonin pharmacological research, because it allows a comparison of melatonin binding sites with responses in a bioassay. Results obtained in binding studies correlate well with physiological responses.[46] In 1995, the melatonin retinal receptor was cloned and found to be of a different subtype than the receptors present in the SCN and the pituitary pars tuberalis.[29] The gene for this new subtype, ML-1b, is not located on the same chromosome as ML-1a, and it is more sensitive to the melatonin antagonist luzindole[1,47] than other melatonin receptor *in vitro* systems.[48,49] The physiological significance of ML-1b in retina is not yet clear, although it is believed that this receptor, along with ML-1a in the CNS, affects circadian and reproductive responses.

In the Cardiovascular System

The most thoroughly studied effect of melatonin on the cardiovascular system is the prolongation and potentiation of noradrenaline-induced contraction of arterial smooth muscle in rat caudal artery.[19] It has been suggested that the rat caudal artery regulates body temperature, and the melatonin binding sites in that vessel may be related to the thermoregulating effect of the hormone. In a study of spontaneously hypertensive rats, which exhibit an impaired ability to dissipate metabolic heat, it was found that the number of receptors was reduced in the caudal artery.[50] Interestingly, reports also imply that the melatonin response is, in some unknown manner, modulated by age and the estrus cycle.[51,52] Autoradiographic studies have shown that the melatonin receptor in rat caudal artery is a high-affinity binding site with a pharmacological profile similar to the profiles of other ML-1 systems.[53] Melatonin binding sites have also been found in part of the circle of Willis,[54] which indicates that melatonin receptors may also be present in other vessels other than the caudal artery.

In Melanophores

The first (and still a most useful) tool in melatonin research is the melanophore, which is a black pigment cell found in the skin of amphibians and fishes. Melatonin induces central aggregation of dispersed pigment granules in melanophores. These cells have been widely used in pharmacological studies ever since Lerner[17] found that melatonin was the "active substance" in his classical experiment on bovine pineal extract. As early as 1969, it was suggested that melatonin could inhibit cAMP levels in frog melanophores,[55] and experiments using different analogs indicated structural demands for efficacy and affinity.[56] Later, methods were developed for culture of melanophores from *Xenopus* embryos,[53] and in 1994 ML-1 receptor cDNA was isolated from an immortalized *Xenopus* melanophore cell line; the pharmacological properties of the receptor were as could be expected for a melatonin receptor.[14] Good correlation was found when comparing melatonin analogs in regard to receptor affinity and potency in inducing pigment aggregation in cultured melanophores, and the *Xenopus* melatonin receptor has been denoted ML-1c.[28]

In the Reproductive System

Although we understand that melatonin plays a role in seasonal reproduction, little is known about where and, in particular, how melatonin interferes with the reproductive system. Some mammals can be categorized as either long-day breeders (e.g., hedgehogs, ferrets, and certain rodents) or short-day breeders (e.g., sheep and deer), depending on whether their gonads are activated by an increasing photoperiod or by a decreasing photoperiod. Melatonin may regulate the timing of reproduction via binding sites in the CNS (probably in the pars tuberalis) and in turn control GnRH secretion.[57,58] Melatonin may also exert a more direct effect, as indicated by the presence of binding sites in both female and male gonads.

Melatonin binding sites have been found in the ovaries of several species, including humans.[59,60] Furthermore, one of the most interesting observations made indicates that melatonin accumulates within human preovulatory fluid, and melatonin binding sites with the affinity and pharmacological profile typical of the ML-1 receptor have been found on human granulosa cell membranes.[61] The melatonin receptors on the granulosa cells are suspected of modulating steroidogenesis, which in turn may be involved in seasonality; hence, the melatonin receptors on the granulosa cells may also mediate a seasonal relationship in human fertility.[36,62] The hormone is now being investigated as a potential contraceptive.[63]

In experiments on rhesus monkeys,[64] parturition usually occurred during hours of darkness, and changing the photoperiod changed the time of birth, as well. Obviously, light seems to have an inhibitory effect on labor. In an *in vitro* study on biopsies from human cesarean sections,[22] the myometrial tissue was mounted in organ baths and allowed to contract spontaneously; subsequent exposure to melatonin was found to augment noradrenaline-induced contractions. The results of binding studies on human myometrium suggest the existence of a binding site with a picomolar affinity for melatonin (Mårtensson, unpublished results), which implicates melatonin binding sites in the timing of human parturition.

Melatonin binding sites, probably ML-1 receptors, have also been found in epithelial cells in benign human prostate tissue. In those experiments, when the prostate epithelial cells were cultured, melatonin was able to inhibit cell growth, perhaps by regulating androgen receptor efficacy (response) or density.[24,65] Further, melatonin binding sites have been detected in the prostatic portion of the rat vas deferens, and melatonin was noted to modulate (through presynaptic regulation) the sympathetic tone in rat vas deferens.[66,67]

In the Immune System

Several investigators have proposed that melatonin can modulate the immune system, but the mechanisms behind this action are not known. Melatonin binding sites have been found in some components of the immune system — for example, in the spleen of different species and in the thymus and the bursa of Fabricius of ducks. Melatonin binding sites have also been observed on circulating human T-lymphocytes,[68] and these sites may mediate an increased release of opioid peptides and interleukin-2, which in turn activate NK cells and antibody-dependent cellular cytotoxicity.[69,70] Notably, mRNA for the ML-1a receptor has not been found in human lymphocytes,[44] which indicates that some other receptor subtype is responsible for the effect mediated by the T-lymphocytes.

In Human Platelets

Del Zar[71,72] found that platelet secretion of adenosine triphosphate (ATP) and serotonin and the production of thromboxane B_2 exhibit a circadian rhythm. In another study, it was found that the profile of the melatonin binding sites on the platelets was similar to the profile of the ML-1 receptor.[73] In contrast to many other investigations, this binding assay of human platelets was done with ^{3}H-melatonin, instead of the more commonly used [^{125}I]melatonin, which may explain the obtained K_d-value of 3 nM. If the binding experiments can be repeated with [^{125}I]melatonin to acquire K_d-values that can be compared with the values obtained for the CNS, it may be possible to use platelets as a model in melatonin research in psychiatry.[74]

Pharmacology and Distribution of the ML-2 Receptor

The ML-2 receptor was identified in binding studies on hamster brain,[2,75] but it has not yet been cloned. The characteristics of the receptor include melatonin affinity in the nanomolar range, faster kinetics, and a pharmacological profile that differs from that of ML-1 — I-melatonin > prazosin (an α_1-adrenoceptor antagonist) $\geq$ N-acetyl-serotonin $\geq$ melatonin.[3] A bioassay has not been developed to study the ML-2 receptor, and ML-2 shows comparatively low affinity for melatonin, thus the significance of this receptor is unknown. In contrast to the ML-1 receptor, the

TABLE 2
Characteristics of 2-[^{125}I]Iodomelatonin Binding Sites

	ML-1	ML-2
Common names	High affinity (pM)	Low affinity (nM)
Affinity states	High (10–300 pM)	High (0.9–10 nM)
	Low (0.3–5 nM)	
Kinetics:		
Association	Slow (t$_{1/2}$ = 9–60 min)	Fast (t$_{1/2}$ = 1–2 min)
Dissociation	Slow (t$_{1/2}$ = <40 min)	Fast (t$_{1/2}$ = 1–2 min)
Regulation:		
GTP	Yes	No
Na$^+$	Yes	No
Ca^{2+}	Yes	No
Mg^{2+}	No	No
Temperature	Yes (affinity increase)	Yes (affinity decrease)
Rank order of affinity	2IMEL	2IMEL
	≥ MEL	> prazosin
	≥ 6-OHMEL	≥ NA5-HT
	>> NA5-HT	≥ 6-OHMEL
	>> prazosin	≥ MEL
	> 5-HT	>> 5-HT
Localization	Retina, SCN, PVNT, SC, PT, AP, CA, CW arteries	Hamster and mouse brain; hamster testes and kidney; RPMI1846 melanoma cells

Note: 2-IMEL = 2-iodomelatonin; MEL = melatonin; 6-OHMEL = 6-hydroxy-melatonin; NA5-HT = N-acetyl-5-hydroxytryptamine; SCN = suprachiasmatic nucleus; PVNT = paraventricular thalamic nucleus; SC = superior colliculus; PT = pars tuberalis; AP = area postrema; CA = caudal artery; CW = circle of Willis.

Source: From Dubocovich, M.L., *Trends Pharmacol. Sci.*, 16, 51, 1995. With permission.

putative ML-2 receptor is not coupled to a G$_i$-protein and it may follow a signal transduction pathway that comprises increased inositol turnover.[76] (For a comparison of ML-1 and ML-2, see Table 2.)

Pharmacology and Distribution of Intracellular Receptors

The first report of melatonin binding, published in 1978, described studies on cytosolic fractions in which a nanomolar level of ^{3}H-melatonin was found to bind specifically to an intracellular receptor.[59] Several years later, in 1994, when the seven transmembrane ML-1 receptor was cloned, Becker-André and Steinhilber[77,78] suggested that melatonin is the natural ligand for an intracellular orphan receptor subfamily referred to as the retinoid Z receptor/retinoid orphan receptor (RZR/RORα-) family. Using [^{125}I]melatonin in transfected HeLa-cells, Becker-André and coworkers found a binding site with a K_d of 5 nM for the RZRβ subtype. RZRβ is expressed only in the brain, and the largest amount of mRNA for the RZRβ receptor is present in the pineal gland.[77] Considering the level of RZRβ mRNA in the pineal and the circadian expression of the protein, as well as the possibility that RZRβ is a melatonin receptor, it has been suggested that RZRβ regulates a negative feedback system for melatonin production in the pineal gland.[79]

Nuclear receptors bind to DNA sequences (response elements) and interact with transcription factors to modulate transcriptional activity. In peripheral tissue, members of the RZR/RORα- family downregulate the expression of 5-lipoxygenase,[78] an enzyme that catalyzes the formation of arachidonic acid into leukotrienes. This could be an example of melatonin-stimulated gene transcription and a link between melatonin and the immune system, especially the inflammatory processes. If this interesting speculation proves true, it may be of significance for the treatment of autoimmune diseases such as rheumatoid arthritis.[80,81]

Melatonin as a Modulating Hormone

It is unclear whether the melatonin binding sites in different systems have a presynaptic or postsynaptic location. For sites modulating neurotransmission release, a presynaptic location has been shown in retina and rat vas deferens; for sites modulating neurotransmission release,[18,67] a postsynaptic location has, for instance, been noted in melanophores[82,83] and rat caudal artery.[19] At present, it is unclear which localization applies to most binding sites.

In some systems, melatonin acts synergistically with noradrenaline. For example, melatonin alone does not induce a response, but it does potentiate a noradrenaline-induced response. Such potentiation can be used to induce smooth muscle contraction in rat caudal artery[19] and human myometrium,[22] and can also be applied to pigment aggregation in melanophores of the cuckoo wrasse, a teleost fish.[6] From a pharmacological perspective, the melatonin response in cuckoo wrasse melanophores seems to be mediated by an α_2-adrenoceptor. By itself, melatonin does not induce pigment aggregation but instead modulates several α_2-adrenoceptor agonists, either by potentiating the action of the agonists, or by acting as an α_2-adrenoceptor antagonist.[6] It is also noteworthy that the α_2-antagonist yohimbine[83] has a far greater effect on the melatonin responses than the melatonin antagonist luzindole does, and that luzindole is also an antagonist of specific α_2-agonists (Mårtensson and Andersson, submitted). Perhaps the effect of melatonin on the melanophore α_2-adrenoceptors is similar to, or occurs in parallel with, described effects on imidazoline binding sites and the α_2-adrenoceptor.

In cuckoo wrasse melanophores, rat caudal artery, and human myometrium, melatonin modulates the sympathetic tone and potentiates noradrenaline-induced action. It has also been shown in melanophores from cuckoo wrasse and a killifish (*Fundulus heteroclitus*)[83,84] that the degree of innervation plays an important role in melatonin-mediated effects.

Conclusions

Melatonin binding sites are most abundant in the brain and in that area have been characterized as ML-1 receptors. The greatest ML-1 density is in the SCN, the location of the biological clock, and in pars tuberalis, which probably controls seasonal coordination of the reproductive system. The highest levels of mRNA for ML-1 have been found to correlate, at least in part, with the binding sites.[30,44,85] Even if the amount of mRNA in the peripheral tissue is low, most of the *in vitro* systems used in melatonin research are based on just such tissues. Therefore, determination and correlation of the location and physiological relevance of melatonin binding sites in parts of the body other than the CNS should become an exciting new area in melatonin research.

It has been suggested that melatonin binding sites are essentially ubiquitous in the bodies of vertebrates, but only a few of the sites have been correlated with a measurable physiological response. This is probably due to the low density of the receptors in peripheral tissues or to the lack of appropriate experimental conditions. In systems in which the action of melatonin can be correlated with a physiological response (e.g., melanophores, rat caudal artery, and rabbit retina), the response is highly influenced by low concentrations (picomolar to nanomolar) of the hormone. Correlation of melatonin binding sites with a physiological response would facilitate understanding of the role of melatonin in the human body. Comprehending the correlation would also allow us to take advantage of the circadian rhythm of melatonin secretion to minimize doses and side effects associated with treatment.

Specific high-affinity antagonists are greatly needed as tools for classification and elucidation of melatonin binding sites. Binding data obtained with agonists can be affected by coupling and uncoupling of G-proteins, which may give spurious K_d and receptor density values. A true antagonist, on the other hand, does not induce any coupling with G-proteins and usually shows higher affinity for receptors. It is also preferable that high-affinity antagonists not be chemically related to melatonin, which would reduce problems with binding to sites that may be regarded as specific receptors but are actually non-receptor sites. The development of specific high-affinity antagonists would make it possible to perform better and more reliable membrane binding studies and would allow further pharmacological characterization of melatonin binding sites *in vitro*. The latter would promote classification of new types or additional subtypes of melatonin receptors.

References

1. Alexander, S.P.H. and Peters, J.A., Receptor and ion channel nomenclature, *Trends Pharmacol. Sci.*, Suppl., 52, 1997.

2. Duncan, M.J., Takahashi, J.S., and Dubocovich, M.L., 2-[^{125}I]Iodomelatonin binding sites in hamster brain membranes: pharmacological characteristics and regional distribution, *Endocrinology*, 122, 1825–1833, 1988.

3. Dubocovich, M.L., Melatonin receptors: are there multiple subtypes?, *Trends Pharmacol. Sci.*, 16, 50–56, 1995.

4. Cohen, M., Roselle, D., and Chabner, B., Evidence for a cytoplasmic melatonin receptor, *Nature*, 274, 894–895, 1978.

5. Carlberg, C. and Wiesenberg, I., The orphan receptor family RZR/ROR, melatonin and 5-lipoxygenase: an unexpected relationship, *J. Pineal Res.*, 18, 171–178, 1995.

6. Mårtensson, L.G.E. and Andersson, R.G.G., A melatonin binding site modulates the α_2-adrenoceptor, *Life Sci.*, 58, 525–533, 1996.

7. Benítez-King, G., Huerto-Delgadillo, L., and Antón-Tay, F., Binding of ^{3}H-melatonin to calmodulin, *Life Sci.*, 53, 201–207, 1993.

8. Bittman, E.L., Melatonin binding sites, *Method. Neurosci.*, 11, 105–120, 1993.

9. Bittman, E.L., The sites and consequences of melatonin binding in mammals, *Am. Zool.*, 33, 200–211, 1993.

10. Kennaway, D.J., Hugel, H.M., and Rowe, S.A., Characterization of the chicken brain melatonin-binding protein using iodonated and tritiated ligands, *J. Pineal Res.*, 17, 137–148, 1994.

11. Swillens, S., Waelbroeck, M., and Champeil, P., Does radiolabelled ligand bind to a homogenous population of non-interacting sites?, *Trends Pharmacol. Sci.*, 16, 151–155, 1995.

12. Bylund, D.B. and Toewes, M.L., Radioligand binding methods: practical guide and tips, *Am. J. Physiol.*, 265, L421–L429, 1993.

13. Kenakin, T., *Pharmacological Analysis of Drug-Receptor Interaction,* Raven Press, New York, 1993.

14. Ebisawa, T., Karne, S., Lerner, M.R., and Reppert, S.M., Expression cloning of a high-affinity melatonin receptor from *Xenopus* dermal melanophores, *Proc. Natl. Acad. Sci. USA*, 91, 6133–6137, 1994.

15. Witt-Enderby, P.A. and Dubocowich, M.L., Characterization and regulation of the human ML-1A melatonin receptor stably expressed in Chinese hamster ovary cells, *Mol. Pharmacol.*, 50, 166–174, 1996.

16. Lefkowitz, R.J., Cotecchia, S., Samana, P., and Costa, T., Constitutive activity of receptors coupled to guanine nucleotide regulatory proteins, *Trends Pharmacol. Sci.*, 14, 303–307, 1993.

17. Lerner, A.B., Case, J.D., Takahashi, Y., Lee, T.H., and Mori, W., Isolation of melatonin, the pineal gland factor that lightens melanocytes, *J. Am. Chem. Soc*, 80, 2567, 1958.

18. Dubocovich, M.L., Melatonin is a potent modulator of dopamine release in the retina, *Nature*, 306, 782–784, 1983.

19. Viswanathan, M., Laitinen, J.T., and Saavedra, J.M., Expression of melatonin receptors in arteries involved in thermoregulation, *Proc. Natl. Acad. Sci. USA*, 87, 6200–6203, 1990.

20. Kornblihtt, L.I., Finocchiaro, L., and Molinas, F.C., Inhibitory effect of melatonin on platelet activation induced by collagen and arachidonic acid, *J. Pineal Res.*, 14, 184–191, 1993.

21. Martín, F.J., Atienza, G., Aldegunde, M., and Míguez, J.M., Melatonin effect on serotonin uptake and release in rat platelets: diurnal variation in responsiveness, *Life Sci.*, 53, 1079–1087, 1993.

22. Mårtensson, L.G.E., Andersson, R.G.G., and Berg, G., Melatonin together with noradrenaline augments contraction of human myometrium., *Eur. J. Pharmacol.*, 316, 273–275, 1996.

23. Ying, S.-W., Niles, L.P., and Crocker, C., Human malignant melanoma cells express high-affinity receptors for melatonin: antiprofilerative effects of melatonin and 6-chloromelatonin., *Eur. J. Pharmacol.*, 246, 89–96, 1993.

24. Gilad, E., Laudon, M., Matzik, H., Pick, E., Sofer, M., Braf, Z., and Zisapel, N., Functional melatonin receptors in human prostrate epithelial cells, *Endocrinology*, 137, 1412–1417, 1996.

25. White, B.H., Sekura, R.D., and Rollag, M.D., Pertussis toxin blocks melatonin-induced pigment aggregation in *Xenopus* dermal melanophores, *J. Comp. Physiol. B*, 157, 153–159, 1987.

26. Fischer, B., Mußhoff, U., Fauteck, J.-D., Madeja, M., Wittkowski, W., and Speckman, E.-J., Expression and functional characterization of melatonin-sensitive receptor in *Xenopus* oocytes, *FEBS Lett.*, 381, 98–102, 1996.

27. Godson, C. and Reppert, S.M., The Mel-1a melatonin receptor is coupled to parallell signal transduction pathways, *Endocrinology,* 138, 397–404, 1997.

28. Reppert, S.M., Weaver, D.R., and Godson, C., Melatonin receptors step into light: cloning and classification of subtypes, *Trends Pharmacol. Sci.*, 17, 100–102, 1996.

29. Reppert, S.M., Godson, C., Mahle, C.D., Weaver, D.R., Slaugenhaupt, S.A., and Gusella, J.F., Molecular characterization of a second melatonin receptor in human retina and brain: the Mel-1b melatonin receptor, *Proc. Natl. Acad. Sci. USA*, 92, 1995.

30. Reppert, S.M., Weaver, D.R., Cassone, V.M., Godson, C., and Kolakowski, J., Melatonin receptors are for the birds: molecular analysis of two receptor subtypes differentially expressed in chicken brain, *Neuron*, 15, 1003–1015, 1995.

31. Masson-Pévet, M., George, D., Kalsbeek, A., Saboureau, M., Lakhdar-Ghazal, N., and Pévet, P., An attempt to correlate brain areas containing melatonin-binding sites with rhythmic functions: a study in five hibernator species, *Cell Tissue Res.*, 278, 97–106, 1994.

32. Gauer, F., Masson-Pévet, M., and Pévet, P., Seasonal regulation of melatonin receptors in rodent pars tuberalis: correlation with reproductive state, *J. Neural Transm.*, 96, 187–195, 1994.

33. Gauer, F., Masson-Pévet, M., Saboureau, M., George, D., and Pévet, P., Differential seasonal regulation of melatonin receptor density in the parstuberalis and in the suprachiasmatic nuclei: a study in the hedgehog (*Erinaceus europaeus, L.*), *J. Neuroendocrinol.*, 5, 685–690, 1993.

34. Nakazawa, K., Marubayashi, U., and McCann, S.M., Mediation of the short-loop negative feedback of luteinizing hormone (LH) on LH-releasing hormone release by melatonin-induced inhibition of LH release from the pars tuberalis, *Proc. Natl. Acad. Sci. USA*, 88, 7576–7579, 1991.

35. Masson-Pévet, M. and Gauer, F., Seasonality and melatonin receptors in the pars tuberalis in some long day breeders, *Biol. Signal.*, 3, 63–70, 1994.

36. Kauppila, A., Kivelä, A., Pakarinen, A., and Vakkuri, O., Inverse seasonal relationship between melatonin and ovarian activity in humans in a region with a strong seasonal contrast in luminosity, *J. Clin. Endocrinol. Metabol.*, 65, 823–828, 1987.

37. Kivelä, A., Kauppila, A., Ylöstalo, P., Vakkuri, O., and Leppäluoto, J., Seasonal, menstrual and circadian secretions of melatonin, gonadotropins and prolactin in women, *Acta Physiol. Scand.,* 132, 321–327, 1988.

38. Rojansky, N., Brzenzinski, A., and Schenker, J.G., Seasonality in human reproduction: an update, *Human Reprod.*, 7, 735–745, 1992.

39. Weaver, D.R., Stehle, J.H., Stopa, E.G., and Reppert, S.M., Melatonin receptors in human hypothalamus and pituitary: implications for circadian and reproductive responses to melatonin, *J. Clin. Endocrinol. Metab.*, 76, 295–301, 1993.

40. Gahr, M. and Kosar, E., Identification, distribution and developmental changes of a melatonin binding site in the song control system of the zebra finch, *J. Comp. Neurol.*, 367, 308–318, 1996.

41. Smith, A., Trudeau, V.L., Williams, L.M., Martinoli, M.-G., and Priede, I.G., Melatonin receptors are present in non-optic regions of the brain of a deep-sea fish living in the absence of solar light, *J. Neroendocrinol.*, 8, 655–658, 1996.

42. Reiter, R.J., Melatonin: the chemical expression of darkness, *Mol. Cell. Endocrinol.,* 79, C153–C158, 1991.

43. Reppert, S.M., Weaver, D.R., and Ebisawa, T., Cloning and characterization of a mammalian melatonin receptor that mediates reproductive and circadian responses, *Neuron,* 13, 1177–1185, 1994.

44. Mazzucchelli, C., Pannacci, M., Nonno, R., Lucini, V., Fraschini, F., and Stankov, B.M., The melatonin receptor in the human brain: cloning experiments and distribution studies, *Mol. Brain Res.*, 39, 117–126, 1996.

45. Gauer, F., Masson-Pevet, M., Stehle, J., and Pévet, P., Daily variations in melatonin receptor density of rat tuberalis and suprachiasmatic nuclei are distinctly regulated, *Brain Res.*, 641, 92–98, 1994.

46. Dubocovich, M.L. and Takahashi, J.S., Use of 2-[^{125}I]iodomelatonin to characterize melatonin binding sites in chicken retina, *Proc. Natl. Acad. Sci. USA,* 84, 3916–3920, 1987.

47. Dubocovich, M.L., Luzindole (N-0774): a novel melatonin antagonist, *J. Pharmacol. Ther.*, 246, 902–910, 1988.

48. Sugden, D., Effect of putative melatonin receptor antagonists on melatonin-induced pigment aggregation in isolated *Xenopus laevis* melanophores, *Eur. J. Pharmacol.*, 213, 405–408, 1992.

49. Krause, D.N., Barrios, V.E., and Piper Duckles, S., Melatonin receptors mediate potentiation of contractile responses to adrenergic nerve stimulation in rat caudal artery, *Eur. J. Pharmacol.*, 276, 207–213, 1995.

50. Viswanathan, M., Laitinen, J.T., and Saavedra, J.M., Differential expression of melatonin receptors in spontaneously hypertensive rats, *Neuroendocrinology*, 56, 864–870, 1992.

51. Seltzer, A., Viswanathan, M., and Saavedra, J.M., Melatonin-binding sites in brain and caudal arteries of the female rat during the estrous cycle and after estrogen administration, *Endocrinology*, 130, 1896–1902, 1992.

52. Laitinen, J.T., Viswanathan, M., Vakkuri, O., and Saavedra, J.M., Differential regulation of the rat melatonin receptors: selective age-associated decline and lack of melatonin-induced changes, *Endocrinology*, 130, 2139–2144, 1992.

53. Viswanathan, M., Laitinen, J.T., and Saavedra, J.M., Vascular melatonin receptors, *Biol. Signals*, 2, 221–227, 1993.

54. Capsoni, S., Viswanathan, M., de Oliveira, A.M., and Saavedra, J.M., Characterization of melatonin receptors and signal transduction system in rat arteries forming the circle of Willis, *Endocrinology*, 135, 373–378, 1994.

55. Abe, K., Robinson, G.A., Liddle, G.W., Butcher, R.W., Nicholson, W.E., and Baird, C.E., Role of cyclic AMP in mediating the effects of MSH, norepinephrine, and melatonin on frog skin color, *Endocrinology*, 85, 674–682, 1969.

56. Heward, C.B. and Hadley, M.E., Structure-activity relationships of melatonin and related indolamines, *Life Sci.*, 17, 1167–1177, 1975.

57. Bartness, T.J., Powers, J.B., Hastings, M.H., Bittman, E.L., and Goldman, B.D., The timed infusion paradigm for melatonin delivery: what has it taught us about the melatonin signal, its reception, and the photoperiodic control of seasonal response?, *J. Pineal. Res.*, 15, 161–190, 1993.

58. Kennaway, D.J. and Rowe, S.A., Melatonin binding sites and their role in seasonal reproduction, *J. Reprod. Fertil.*, Suppl. 49, 423–435, 1995.

59. Cohen, M., Roselle, D., and Chabner, B., Evidence for a cytoplasmic melatonin receptor, *Nature,* 274, 894–895, 1978.

60. Ayre, E.A. and Pang, S.F., 2-[^{125}I]Iodomelatonin binding sites in the testis and ovary: putative melatonin receptors in the gonads, *Biol. Signals*, 3, 71–84, 1994.

61. Yie, S.-M., Niles, L.P., and Younglai, E.V., Melatonin receptors on human granulosa cell membranes, *J. Clin. Endocr. Metab.*, 80, 1747–1749, 1995.

62. Yie, S.-M., Brown, G.M., Liu, G.-Y., Collins, J.A., Daya, S., Hughes, E.G., Foster, W.G., and Younglai, E.V., Melatonin and steroids in human pre-ovulatory follicular fluid: seasonal variations and granulosa cell steroid production, *Hum. Reprod.*, 10, 50–55, 1995.

63. Silman, R.E., Melatonin: a contraceptive for the nineties, *Eur. J. Obstet. R.P.*, 49, 3–9, 1993.

64. Ducsay, C.H. and Yellon, S.M., Photoperiod regulation of uterine activity and mela-tonin rhythms in the pregnant rhesus macaque, *Biol. Reprod.*, 44, 967–974, 1991.

65. Laudon, M., Gilad, E., Matzkin, H., Braf, Z., and Zisapel, N., Putative melatonin receptors in benign human prostrate tissue, *J. Clin. Endocrinol. Metab.*, 81, 1336–1342, 1996.

66. Carneiro, R.C.G., Markus, R.P., and Dubocovich, M.L., 2-[125I]Iodomelatonin bind-ing sites in the rat vas deferens, *Biol. Signals*, 2, 194–198, 1993.

67. Carneiro, R.C.G., Markus, R.P., and Dubocovich, M.L., Presynaptic modulation by melatonin of the nicotine-induced calcium-dependent release of norepinephrine from rat vas deferens, *Biol. Signals*, 2, 199–206, 1993.

68. Gonzalez-Haba, M.G., Garcia-Mauriño, S., Calvo, J.R., Goberna, R., and Guerrero, J.M., High-affinity binding of melatonin by human circulating T lymphocytes (CD4+), *FASEB J.*, 9, 1331–1335, 1995.

69. Giordano, M., Vermeulen, M., and Palermo, M., Seasonal variations in antibody-dependent cellular cytotoxicity regulation by melatonin, *FASEB J.*, 7, 1052–1054, 1993.

70. Guerro, J.M. and Reiter, R.J., A brief survey of pineal gland-immune system interre-lationships, *Endocr. Res.*, 18, 91–113, 1992.

71. Del Zar, M.M., Martinuzzo, M., Cardinali, D.P., Carreras, L.O., and Vacas, M.I., Diurnal variation in melatonin effect on adenosine triphosphate and serotonin release by human platelets, *Acta Endocrinol.*, 123, 453–458, 1990.

72. Del Zar, M.M., Martinuzzo, M., Falcón, C., Cardinali, D.P., Carreras, L.O., and Vacas, M.I., Inhibition of human platelet aggregation and thromboxane-B₂ production by melatonin: evidence for a diurnal variation, *J. Clin. Endocrinol. Metabol.*, 70, 246–251, 1990.

73. Vacas, M.I., Del Zar, M.M., Martinuzzo, M., and Cardinali, D.P., Binding sites for [3H]-melatonin in human platelets, *J. Pineal Res.*, 13, 60–65, 1992.

74. Wahlund, B., Sääf, J., and Wetterberg, L., Classification of patients with affective disorders using platelet monoamine oxidase activity, serum melatonin and post-dexamethasone cortisol, *Acta Psychiatr. Scand.*, 91, 313–321, 1995.

75. Niles, L.P., Pickering, D.S., and Sayer, B.G., HPLC-purified 2-[125I]iodomelatonin labels multiple binding sites in hamster brain, *Biochem. Biophys. Res. Co.*, 147, 949–956, 1987.

76. Eison, A.S. and Mullins, U.L., Melatonin binding sites are functionally coupled to phosphoinositide hydrolysis in syrian hamster RPMI 1846 melanoma cells, *Life Sci.*, 53, PL393–398, 1993.

77. Becker-André, M., Wiesenberg, I., Schaeren-Wiemers, N., André, E., Missbach, M., Saurat, J.-H., and Carlberg, C., Pineal gland hormone melatonin binds and activates an orphan of the nuclear receptor superfamily, *J. Biol. Chem.*, 269, 28531–28534, 1994.

78. Steinhilber, D., Brungs, M., Werz, O., Wiesenberg, I., Danielsson, C., Kahlen, J.-P., Nayeri, S., Schräder, M., and Carlberg, C., The nuclear receptor for melatonin represses 5-lipoxygenase gene expression in human B lymphocytes, *J. Biol. Chem.*, 270, 7037–7040, 1995.

79. Baler, R., Coon, S., and Klein, D.C., Orphan nuclear receptor RZRβ: cyclic AMP regulates expression in the pineal gland, *Biochem. Biophys. Res*, 220, 975–978, 1996.

80. Carlberg, C. and Wiesenberg, I., The orphan receptor family RZR/ROR, melatonin and 5-lipoxygenase: an unexpected relationship, *J. Pineal Res.*, 18, 171–178, 1995.

81. Missbach, M., Jagher, B., Sigg, I., Nayeri, S., Carlberg, C., and Wiesenberg, I., Thiazolidine diones, specific ligands of the nuclear receptor retinoid Z receptor/ retonoid acid receptor-related orphan receptor α with potent antiarthritic activity, *J. Biol. Chem.*, 271, 13515–13522, 1996.

82. Messenger, E.A. and Warner, A.E., The action of melatonin on single amphibian pigment cells in tissue culture, *Br. J. Pharmacol.,* 61, 607–614, 1977.

83. Mårtensson, L.G.E. and Andersson, R.G.G., Denervation of pigment cells lead to a receptor that is ultrasensitive for melatonin and noradrenaline, *Life Sci.*, 60, 1575–1582, 1997.

84. Fain, W.B. and Hadley, M.E., *In vitro* response of melanophores of *Fundulus heteroclitus* to melatonin, adrenaline and noradrenaline, *Am. Zool.*, 6, 596, 1966.

85. Mazzucchelli, C., Capsoni, S., Angeloni, D., Fraschini, F., and Stankov, B., Expression of the melatonin receptor in *Xenopus laevis*: a comparative study between protein and mRNA distribution, *J. Pineal Res.*, 20, 57–64, 1996.

Chapter **2**

Localization and Physiological Significance of Gastrointestinal Melatonin

George A. Bubenik

Contents

Introduction

What is melatonin and why has so much been written in recent years about its effects on various body systems? Melatonin is a remarkable chemical which is partly a hormone (effective in humans at incredibly low concentrations of three tenths of a thousandth of a gram),[1] and partly a vitamin-like compound, effective as an antioxidant.[2] In both capacities, melatonin seems to enjoy a promising future as a therapeutic

0-8493-8564-4/99/$0.00+$.50
© 1999 by CRC Press LLC

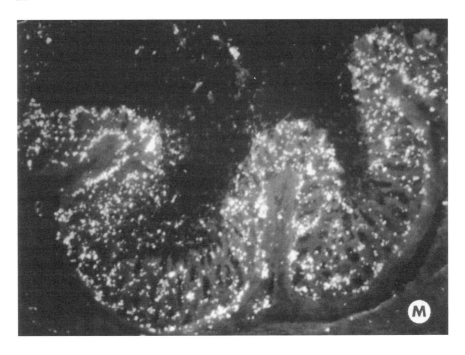

FIGURE 1

Histological localization of melatonin in the rat colon using immunofluorescence. Note that most melatonin is located in the mucosa and not in the muscularis (M).

or prophylactic medicine[3] and has therefore generated enormous interest of the scientific and popular press.

Melatonin is an evolutionary relict, an ubiquitous molecule preserved in diverse species for at least 3.5 billion years. It was recently detected in unicellular microorganisms and algaes; in numerous plants and invertebrates such as insects, worms, and crustaceans; and in all vertebrates.[4] After the discovery of melatonin by Aaron Lerner and his co-workers in 1958,[5] it was generally believed, that this chemical is produced only in the pineal gland.[6] Only in the 1970s did reports of extrapineal localization of melatonin and indications of its production in diverse body tissues such as the retina, Harderian gland, and the gastrointestinal tract (GIT; see Figure 1)[7–11] result in the acceptance of extrapineal sources of melatonin.[12]

Location, Production Sites, and Physiological Functions

Whereas research on melatonin in the retina and the Harderian gland gained speed in the 1980s, there was very little interest in investigations of melatonin in the GIT. This was unfortunate, because the vertebrate GIT is a major source of melatonin

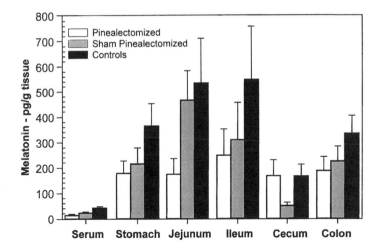

FIGURE 2

Melatonin concentration in serum and GIT tissues of control, sham-pinealectomized, and pinealectomized rats sacrificed at midnight. (From Bubenik, G.A. and Brown, G.M., *Biol. Signals*, 195, 40, 1997. With permission.)

production. According to the calculations of Huether,[13] there is at least 400× more melatonin in the GIT of birds and mammals than in their pineal glands. In addition, in all species so far investigated, including the lower vertebrates,[14] melatonin levels in GIT tissue have exceeded their levels in plasma by 5 to 10 times (Figure 2).[15-20] Despite these astonishing findings, very few scientists devoted their long-term effort to study GIT melatonin. Only recently has a growing interest in this area of melatonin research emerged,[21-23] particularly with respect to the potential clinical utilization of this remarkable compound.[24]

The delay in the investigations of GIT melatonin was regrettable, because a quick start in this area of research could have fostered rapid progress. Just 7 years after the discovery of melatonin,[3] Quastel and Rahamimoff[25] observed the distinct effect of this indole on the peristalsis of the rat duodenum. This initial study was followed by reports of a strong antiserotonin action of melatonin when used in the rat stomach and ileum.[26,27] This effect of melatonin as a natural inhibitor of serotonin action in the GIT and its influence on muscle tone were later confirmed by Bubenik[28] (Figure 3) and Harlow and Weekly[29] *in vitro*. In their studies, melatonin was shown to relax smooth muscles of the GIT and to counteract the spastic effect of serotonin. In later *in vivo* studies, melatonin increased the food transit time which had been shortened in mice previously implanted with serotonin-containing pellets (Figure 4).[30] A decade after the pioneering study of Quastel and Rahamimoff,[25] a Russian group lead by Raikhlin detected melatonin in the human appendix using paper chromatography.[31] Later, using a histochemical technique, they concluded that melatonin is most probably produced in the enterochromaffin cells of the GIT mucosa.[31-33] Shortly afterward, using newly developed antibodies specific against

A

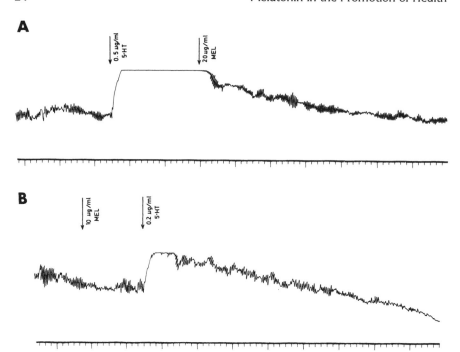

B

FIGURE 3
The effect of melatonin on the function of rat ileum *in vitro*. (**A**) Melatonin treatment relieved the serotonin-induced spasm and restarted the peristalsis. (**B**) Pretreatment with melatonin prevented a subsequent spasm induced by serotonin. (From Bubenik, G.A., *J. Pineal Res.*, 3, 41, 1986. With permission.)

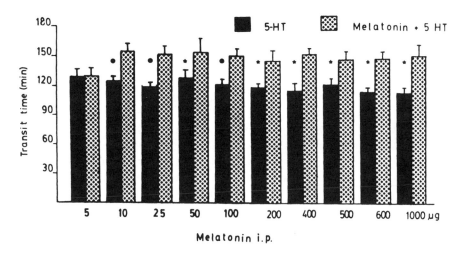

FIGURE 4
The effect of various doses of melatonin on the food transit time of mice bearing implants of 2 mg of serotonin. Mice were injected intraperitoneally with melatonin 50 min after being fed. * = $p < 0.05$; • = $p < 0.01$. (From Bubenik, G.A. and Dhanvantari, S., *J. Pineal Res.*, 7, 333, 1989. With permission.)

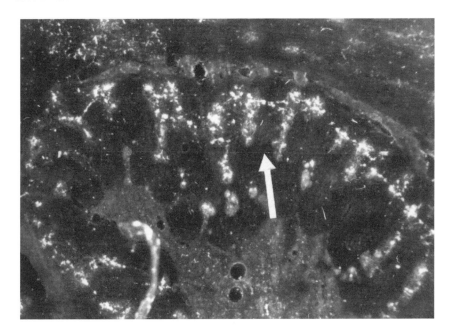

FIGURE 5
Immunohistological localization of melatonin in the mucosa of the rat colon. Fluorescence indicates the presence of melatonin in the deeper segments of Lieberkuhn crypts (arrow). (From Brown, G.M. et al., *Adv. Biosci.,* 29, 95, 1980. With permission.)

melatonin,[34] this indole was localized immunohistologically in the mucosa of the entire rat GIT, ranging from esophagus to rectum (Figure 5).[10] Such distribution of melatonin was confirmed a few years later by Holloway and co-workers.[35]

Pineal and Extrapineal Sources of Melatonin

Whereas the presence of melatonin in the GIT was confirmed by various techniques, this still did not prove that melatonin is produced in these tissues; therefore, the detection in the GIT tissues of the two enzymes, hydroxyindole-O-methyltransferase[36] and N-acetyltransferase,[37] which are involved in melatonin synthesis, was crucial for the acceptance of melatonin production.

In intact animals, circadian levels of melatonin in blood are photoperiodically regulated, resulting in a rapid increase of their levels after the onset of darkness. It has been established that the several-fold increase of melatonin in blood during the night is due to a rapid production and immediate secretion of melatonin from the pineal gland.[38] A similar circadian variation of melatonin levels, independent of the pineal, was also observed in the retina.[39] However, GIT melatonin differs from melatonin produced in these two other extrapineal sources. The independent nature of melatonin production in the GIT was first revealed in 1980, when it was found that

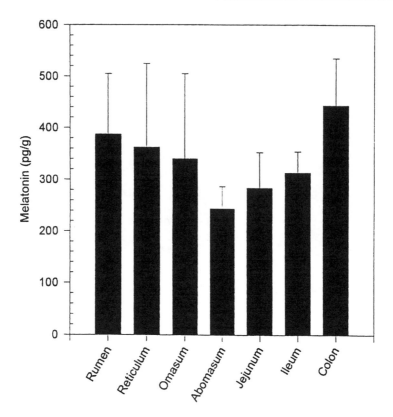

FIGURE 6
Melatonin in fetal calves during the second trimester of pregnancy.

pinealectomy (the removal of the pineal gland) does not reduce the amount of melatonin in the digestive tract. In addition, contrary to plasma, no diurnal variations of melatonin levels were found in most GIT tissues.[15,16,41] In addition, unlike in the pineal gland where melatonin production in rats begins only one week postnatally,[42] melatonin was already localized in the GIT of perinatal rats.[40,43] Most recently, very high concentrations of melatonin (250 to 300 pg/g tissue) were detected in all GIT segments of fetal calves, obtained during the second trimester of pregnancy (Figure 6).[44] Finally, melatonin was also detected in the GIT of chicken embryos,[20] thus indicating that GIT production is independent of maternal circulation.

In the mid 1980s, melatonin was finally detected by radioimmunoassay in the GIT of pigeons, where no diurnal variation of melatonin levels was also observed in most tissues, except duodenum.[41] The lack of diurnal variations in melatonin levels in most GIT tissues was later also confirmed in mice (Figure 7),[45] ducks,[46] and chicken embryos.[20] The detection of melatonin in the GIT tissues after pinealectomy (Figure 2)[15,40] supported its independent secretion throughout the digestive system.

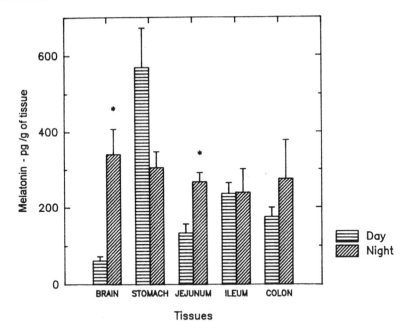

FIGURE 7
Melatonin in the brain and GIT of mice sacrificed at midday and at midnight. * indicates significantly higher levels ($p < 0.05$). (From Bubenik, G.A. et al., *Comp. Biochem. Physiol.*, 104C, 221, 1993. With permission.)

Contribution of GIT to Melatonin in Systemic Circulation

In the early studies, the sensitivity of detection assays was so low that the removal of the pineal gland resulted in non-detectable levels of melatonin in blood. That supported the hypothesis that the pineal gland is the sole producer of melatonin;[6,47] however, as melatonin assays became more sensitive, a different picture emerged. In numerous newer studies, which used radioimmunoassays and gas chromatography, pinealectomy abolished only the nighttime elevation of melatonin in plasma,[48] but substantial daytime levels were still present. Interestingly, these basal levels persisted as long as the rats were fed the *ad libitum* diet but disappeared when food was restricted.[47] In retrospect, that observation indicated that melatonin in pinealectomized animals is of GIT origin and its secretion related to food intake. In birds and mammals, the digestive system was the only viable source of that extrapineal melatonin because the removal of the retina or the Harderian gland, the other two extrapineal sources of melatonin, did not alter daytime levels of melatonin in blood.[49] The only exception was found in lower vertebrates; in fish, removal of both eyes significantly reduced plasma levels of melatonin in pinealectomized animals.[49,50] Whereas an independent GIT secretion was firmly established a few years ago, it was generally believed that GIT melatonin acts mostly locally in a paracrine fashion.[23] That changed when an intriguing hypothesis emerged which speculated that a substantial amount of melatonin produced in the GIT in response to feeding finds its way into the peripheral circulation.[10,51–53] Some earlier studies indicated a possible role of food intake in the regulation of diurnal rhytmicity. More than 20 years ago, Krieger and co-workers reported that diurnal rhythms of temperature, locomotion, and cortisol in blood was shifted in rats by food presentation.[54] That periodic feeding can act as a zeitgeber of various biological rhythms was confirmed by Ho and co-workers.[55] In retrospect, it can be speculated, that the shift of biological rhythms might have been induced by a temporary increase of peripheral levels of melatonin originating in the GIT in response to feeding.

As was stated earlier, the presence of melatonin in pinealectomized animals indicated that extrapineal production sites, most probably in the GIT,[46,48] are the source of daytime levels of peripheral melatonin. However, the presence of melatonin in blood after pinealectomy was not sufficient proof that melatonin produced in the GIT is secreted into systemic circulation. The elegant studies by Huether and co-workers definitely confirmed that GIT is a source of melatonin in the peripheral blood. In the first study, daytime oral administration of L-tryptophan, the amino acid precursor of melatonin, substantially increased melatonin levels in the peripheral blood of humans.[51] A fourfold increase of melatonin after administration of tryptophan was detected in the rat portal vein, the blood vessel which brings nutrient-rich blood from the GIT to liver.[52] Furthermore, tryptophan administration elevated peripheral blood levels of melatonin twofold in pinealectomized rats,[52,53] thus demonstrating that extrapineal tissues are the source of the peripheral melatonin elevation. Finally, the GIT origin of melatonin elevation in the systemic blood after food intake was clearly demonstrated when the increase of melatonin levels in the peripheral circulation observed in pinealectomized rats was prevented by a ligation of the portal vein.[51] Based on these facts, it was postulated that the profound nocturnal elevation of melatonin in plasma of vertebrate species is due to its production in the pineal gland; however, the steady basal levels of melatonin seen during the daytime may originate in the GIT.[13]

Melatonin and Food Intake

Increasing evidence indicates a relationship between the concentration of GIT melatonin and food intake. Melatonin implants altered the amount of food consumed by mice.[43] Several other studies reported that re-feeding of animals after a period of fasting will temporarily elevate melatonin levels in blood (Figure 8).[17,19,56] A similar increase of melatonin after an evening meal was also observed in human saliva.[57] This rapid rise of melatonin levels in the peripheral blood after re-feeding may constitute the pulse which may have caused the previously mentioned shift in biological rhythms, including locomotion, temperature, and cortisol rhythm, observed by Krieger and co-workers.[54]

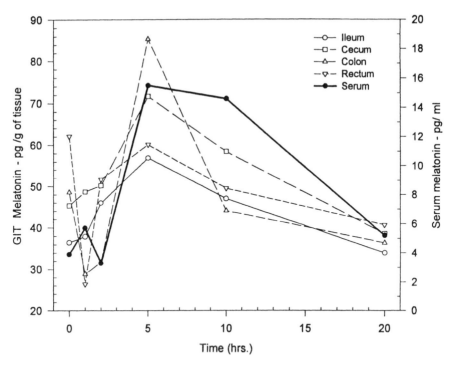

FIGURE 8

Melatonin levels in serum and GIT tissues of pigs fasted for 30 hr and then sacrificed at 1, 2, 5, 10, and 20 hr after re-feeding. Note the synchrony of melatonin increase in serum and GIT tissues. (From Bubenik, G.A. et al., *J. Pineal Res.*, 21, 251, 1996. With permission.)

As was mentioned earlier, the levels of GIT melatonin are related to nutritional condition, particularly food supply. Several studies, performed primarily in the 1980s and 1990s, investigated the effect of food intake on melatonin levels in the pineal gland, peripheral blood, and the GIT tissues. A reduction in food intake had a significant effect on pineal activity and serum melatonin levels. In rats, long-term reduction in food intake decreased melatonin levels in the pineal by 12%;[58] however, serum melatonin levels of food-restricted rats increased by 34%.[59] Underfeeding has also been shown to elevate daytime levels of melatonin in pigs[60] as well as to increase daytime levels of melatonin in serum of human volunteers.[61] In addition, higher melatonin levels were reported in blood of human patients suffering from anorexia nervosa, a mental disorder characterized by a severe voluntary restriction of food intake.[62] A long-term fasting substantially elevated melatonin levels in GIT tissues of mammals[16,19] and birds.[22] Interestingly, an inhibition of melatonin elevation observed in humans after short-term fasting[63] was reversed by an oral administration of glucose.[64]

The discrepancy between pineal and plasma levels of melatonin after fasting could be explained by a simultaneous decrease of melatonin synthesis in the pineal gland and an increase in melatonin production in the GIT which spills over into the peripheral circulation. However, as very little is known about the relationship of the pineal gland and the GIT, more studies are necessary to elucidate the possibility of the existence of such feedback mechanism.

The temporary increase of plasma melatonin levels after re-feeding correlated with the elevation of melatonin in the tissues of the lower GIT; therefore, it was speculated that the origin of melatonin elevation observed in the systemic circulation after food intake is in the lower segments of the GIT.[17] What could be the physiological significance of such a phenomenon? Perhaps melatonin modulates the digestive functions not only via its action at the smooth muscles[28] but also via the central nervous system (CNS), as has been recently suggested.[65,66] In that function, melatonin could be involved in the CNS regulation of food intake[43] or in the synchronization of feeding and digestive processes.[17]

Does Pineal Melatonin Contribute to Melatonin in the GIT?

Whereas it is now certain that not all melatonin in peripheral circulation is of pineal origin, not all melatonin detected in the GIT tissues might be produced in the digestive system. Some of the gut melatonin might be of extrinsic origin; a massive uptake of melatonin in the GIT tissues was reported after administration of exogenous melatonin.[40,56,67,68] It was therefore speculated that perhaps the higher nocturnal levels of melatonin observed in some GIT tissues[16,41] might be due to the uptake of melatonin produced in the pineal gland during the night.[40] The possibility of nighttime binding of melatonin in the GIT tissue was strengthened by the detection of GIT melatonin binding sites. These binding sites, which mostly exhibited diurnal variation, were detected in GIT tissues of birds[22] and mammals,[45] including humans.[69,70] In ducks, the binding sites were detected as early as 5 days before hatching,[23] thus indicating the functional significance of melatonin during fetal development.

Melatonin and Gastrointestinal Diseases

Gastric Ulcers

The early studies of Quastel and Rahamimoff,[25] Fioretti et al.,[26,27] and Bubenik[28] indicated that melatonin may act as a physiological inhibitor of serotonin (5-hydroxytryptamine, or 5-HT) in visceral smooth muscles,[16] acting probably as a competitive agonist of 5-HT inhibitory receptors.[28] Melatonin restored the motility of rat intestine after serotonin-induced spasm[28] and extended the food transit time previously reduced by 5-HT.[31] In addition, melatonin administration reversed the serotonin-induced reduction of blood flow and decreased the incidence of ethanol-induced gastric ulcers.[71] In rats, melatonin prevented stress-induced gastric lesions, presumably by counteracting the serotonin-induced reduction in blood flow.[72] Recently, a minute amount of melatonin administered through food (2.5 mg/kg of food) reduced the incidence and severity of gastric ulcers in pigs.[73] Another study in pigs revealed that animals with the most severe ulcers exhibited significantly lower levels of melatonin in serum and stomach tissues. In addition, pigs fed a coarsely ground diet exhibited significantly higher levels of melatonin in their stomach tissues than animals fed a finely ground diet. No such relationships were found for other parts of the GIT.[18] Finally, melatonin was reported to protect the gastric mucosa from lesions induced by a severe stress[74,75] or by ischemia and reperfusion.[74] The mechanisms of the protective action of melatonin in the gastric mucosa was ascribed to the diminution in the production of free radicals, the stimulation of secretion of prostaglandins, and the increase in gastric blood flow.[75]

The above studies indicate that perhaps the gastroprotective effect of a coarsely ground diet is mediated by melatonin produced in the gastric mucosa. In addition, it could be hypothesized that the aspirin-induced inflammation of the gastric mucosa could be counteracted by a simultaneous administration of small doses of melatonin.

Colitis

Recently, Bubenik and Pang[43] postulated a mutual melatonin-serotonin feedback which secures a proper balance between stimulatory and inhibitory actions in the GIT. In addition to the stomach, another GIT tissue — colon — may be affected by the imbalance between these two closely related indoles. Overproduction of 5-HT speeds colonic transit time[30] and causes diarrhea and ulceration.[76] Melatonin counteracts these undesirable effects of 5-HT, as was recently demonstrated by Pentney and Bubenik.[77] Daily administration of melatonin eliminated most symptoms of experimentally induced colitis in mice. Rectal bleeding, occult blood in feces, loss of weight, and focal lesions of colonic mucosa induced by dextran sodium sulfate (DSS) were almost entirely eliminated after several weeks of treatment (Figure 9). Interestingly, serum levels of melatonin in mice treated with DSS were more than 10 times higher than levels in controls.

The authors concluded that the remarkable improvement in the conditions of melatonin-treated mice might be due to its capacity as an antioxidant[2] or due to its effect on the immune system of the gut.[78,79] Another contributing factor might be the stimulatory effect of melatonin on the mitotic activity observed in the mice intestinal epithelium.[80] Furthermore, melatonin may have alleviate the diarrhea by altering the movement of fluids across the intestinal wall. In rat colon, melatonin inhibited amiloride-sensitive epithelial sodium absorption.[81] Finally, the finding of the substantial elevation of serum levels of melatonin in DSS-treated mice might have been caused by an increased production of melatonin in the GIT (stimulated by the inflammation) which subsequently resulted in an elevation of melatonin in the systemic circulation. If this was the case in the colitis study, then the Raihklin group made a lucky choice more than 20 years ago when they decided to use an inflamed appendix for their first chromatographical detection of GIT melatonin.[31] However,

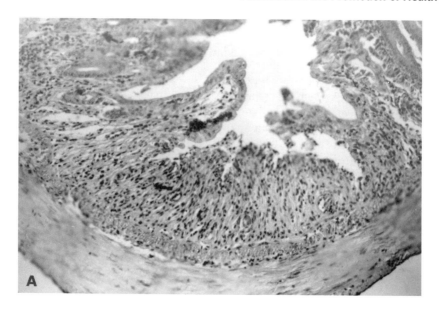

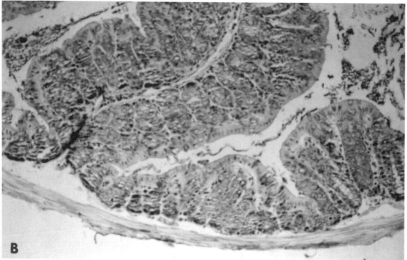

FIGURE 9

(A) Erosive lesions of mucosa in colon of mice with colitis induced with dextran sodium sulfate (DSS). Sections show a heavy lymphocyte infiltration and focal disappearance of crypts. (B) Mucosa of mice receiving DSS and treated with melatonin. Note the almost complete recovery of all layers of mucosa. (From Pentney, P. and Bubenik, G.A., *J. Pin. Res.*, 19, 31, 1995. With permission.)

because experimental evidence is not yet available, only future studies of the GIT immune system might elucidate the role melatonin plays in the prevention of gastrointestinal diseases such as colitis.

Cancer

The relationship between melatonin and cancer is discussed in Chapter 4. Nevertheless, it is interesting to note that Kvetnoy and Levin[82] reported a reversal of diurnal levels of urine melatonin (higher during the day and lower during the night) in patients suffering from gastric and rectal cancer. As the total amount of melatonin excreted over a 24-hr period was not different from the control group, it was speculated that in cancer patients melatonin produced in extrapineal sources alters the rhythm of melatonin synthesis in the pineal gland.[68] However, these findings were not confirmed by a recent study of Vician and co-workers[83] in patients suffering from colon cancer, where higher melatonin levels in plasma and saliva were found during the night. In addition, melatonin was found to be only a weak antagonist of mitosis of human colon cancer cells maintained *in vitro*.[84] In view of these discrepancies, more studies are necessary to reveal any possible relationship between melatonin and GIT malignancies.

Colic

As possible natural inhibitors of serotonin, melatonin and 5-HT may maintain a mutual balance.[43] Disruption of the serotonin-melatonin balance might cause the painful abdominal affliction known as a colic. As colics are observed mostly in young children, in which melatonin levels are relatively low, Weissbluth and Weissbluth[85] speculated that the imbalance between the melatonin and 5-HT is a cause of the pain and abdominal discomfort characterizing colic. Once the melatonin levels reach a balance with 5-HT, which is at about 3 months of age, most colics disappear.

Summary

Mucosa of the gastrointestinal tract is a major production site of melatonin, accounting for most of the daytime levels detected in the peripheral circulation. The GIT melatonin secretion, stimulated by food intake, can result in the elevation of melatonin levels in the systemic circulation. Conversely, during the nighttime, melatonin of pineal origin can bind to binding sites detected in the mucosa. There are prospects of clinical utilization of melatonin for treatment of GIT disorders, such as gastric ulcers, colitis, and cancer. The mechanism of melatonin action in the GIT may include scavenging of free radicals, stimulation of the immune system, and the transmembrane movement of fluids.

References

1. Zhdanova, I.V., Wurtman, R.J., Lynch, H.J., Yves, J.R., Dollins, A.B., Morabito, C., Matheson, J.K., and Schomer, D.L., Sleep-inducing effects of low doses of melatonin ingested in the evening, *Clin. Pharmacol. Ther.*, 57, 552, 1995.

2. Reiter, R.J., Tang L., Garcia, J.J., and Munoz-Hoyos, A., Pharmacological actions of melatonin in oxygen radical pathophysiology, *Life Sci.,* 60, 2255, 1997.

3. Reiter, R.J. and Robinson. J., *Melatonin,* Bantam Press, New York, 1995, 1–291.

4. Hardeland, R. and Fuhrberg, B., Ubiquitous melatonin — presence and effects in unicells, plants and animals. *Trends Comp. Biochem. Physiol.,* 2, 25, 1996.

5. Lerner, A.A., Case, J.D., Takahashi, Y., Lee, T.H., and Mori, W., Isolation of melatonin, the pineal factor that lightens melanocytes. *J. Am. Chem. Soc.,* 80, 33, 1958.

6. Wurtman, R.J., Axelrod, J., and Kelly, D., *The Pineal,* Academic Press, New York, 1968.

7. Cardinali, D.P. and Wurtman, R.J., Hydroxyindole-*O*-methyltransferase in rat pineal, retina, and the Harderian gland, *Endocrinology* 91, 247, 1972.

8. Bubenik, G.A., Uhlir, I., Brown, G.M., and Grota, L.J., Immunohistological localization of acetylindolealkylamines in pineal gland, retina and cerebellum, *Brain Res.,* 81, 233, 1974.

9. Bubenik, G.A., Brown, G.M., and Grota, L.J., Differential localization of *N*-acetylated indolealkylamines in the CNS and the Harderian gland, *Brain Res.* 118, 417, 1976.

10. Bubenik, G.A., Brown, G.M., and Grota, L.J., Immunohistological localization of melatonin in the rat digestive tract, *Experientia* 33, 662, 1977.

11. Pang, S.F., Brown, G.M., Grota, L.J., Chambers, J.W., and Rodman, R.L., Determination of *N*-acetylserotonin and melatonin activities in the pineal gland, retina, Harderian gland, brain and serum of rats and chickens, *Neuroendocrinology,* 23, 1, 1977.

12. Ralph, C.L., Melatonin production by extrapineal tissues, *Adv. Biosci.,* 29, 35, 1981.

13. Huether, G., The contribution of extrapineal sites of melatonin synthesis to circulating melatonin levels in higher vertebrates, *Experientia,* 49, 665, 1993.

14. Bubenik, G.A. and Pang, S.F., Melatonin in the gastrointestinal tissues of fish, amphibians, and a reptile, *Gen. Comp. Endocrinol.,* 106, 415, 1997.

15. Bubenik, G.A. and Brown, G.M., Pinealectomy reduces melatonin levels in serum but not in the gastrointestinal tract of the rat, *Biol. Signals,* 195, 40, 1997.

16. Bubenik, G.A. Ball, R.O., and Pang, S.F., The effect of food deprivation on brain and gastrointestinal tissue levels of tryptophan, serotonin, 5-hydroxyindoleacetic acid, and melatonin, *J. Pineal Res.,* 12, 7, 1992.

17. Bubenik, G.A., Pang, S.F., Hacker, R.R., and Smith, P.S., Melatonin concentrations in serum and tissues of porcine gastrointestinal tract and their relationship to the intake and passage of food, *J.Pineal Res.,* 21, 251, 1996.

18. Bubenik, G.A., Ayles, H.L., Friendship, R.M., Brown, G.M., and Ball, R.O., Relationship between melatonin levels in plasma and gastrointestinal tissues and the incidence and severity of gastric ulcers in pigs, *J. Pineal Res.,* 24, 62–66, 1997.

19. Huether, G., Melatonin synthesis in the gastrointestinal tract and the impact of nutritional factors on circulating melatonin, *Ann. N.Y. Acad. Sci.,* 719, 146, 1994.

20. Zeman, M., Embryonic and early postembryonic development of rhythmic melatonin production in the pineal gland, retina and gut of birds, presented at 5th Canadian Pineal and Melatonin Symposium, Guelph, July 13 to 15, 1997.

21. Lee, P.P.N., Hong, G.X., and Pang, S.F., Melatonin in the gastrointestinal tract, in Fraschini, F. and Reiter, R.J., Eds., *Role of Melatonin and Pineal Peptides in Neuroimmodulation,* Plenum Press, New York, 1991, 127.

22. Lee, P.P.N. and Pang, S.F., Melatonin and its receptors in the gastrointestinal tract, *Biol. Signals,* 2, 181, 1993.

23. Chow, P.H., Lee, P.N., Poon, A.M.S., Shiu, S.Y.W., and Pang, S.F., The gastrointestinal system: a site of melatonin paracrine action, in Tang, P.L., Pang, S.F., and Reiter, R.J., Eds., *Frontiers of Hormone Research,* Vol. 21, *Melatonin: A Universal Photoperiodic Signal with Diverse Action,* Basel, Karger, 1996, 123.

24. Maestroni, J.M. and Reiter, R.J., *Frontiers of Hormone Research,* Vol. 23, *Therapeutic Potential of Melatonin,* Basel, Karger, 1997, 1.

25. Quastel, M.R. and Rahamimoff R., Effect of melatonin on spontaneous contraction and response to 5-hydroxytryptamine of rat isolated duodenum, *Br. J. Pharmacol.,* 24, 455, 1965.

26. Fioretti, M.C., Barzi, F., and Martini, L., Affinity of melatonin for serotonin receptors in the isolated rat stomach, *Riv. Farmacol. Terap.,* 3, 383, 1972 (in Italian).

27. Fioretti, M.C., Menconi, E., and Riccardi, C., Mechanisms of the *in vitro* 5-hydroxytryptamine (5-HT) antagonism exerted by pineal indole derivatives, *Riv. Farmacol. Terap.,* 5, 43, 1974 (in Italian).

28. Bubenik, G.A., The effect of serotonin, *N*-acetylserotonin, and melatonin on spontaneous contractions of isolated rat intestine, *J. Pineal Res.,* 3, 41, 1986.

29. Harlow, H.J. and Weekly, B.L., Effect of melatonin on the force of spontaneous contractions of *in vitro* rat small and large intestine, *J. Pineal Res.,* 3, 277, 1986.

30. Bubenik, G.A. and Dhanvantari, S., The influence of serotonin and melatonin on some parameters of gastrointestinal activity, *J. Pineal Res.,* 7, 333, 1989.

31. Raikhlin, N.T., Kvetnoy, I.M., and Tolkachev, V.N., Melatonin may be synthesized in enterochromaffin cells, *Nature,* 255, 344, 1975.

32. Raikhlin N.T. and Kvetnoy I.M., Melatonin and enterochromaffin cells, *Acta Histochem.,* 55, 19, 1976.

33. Raikhlin, N.T., Kvetnoy, I.M., Kadagidze, Z.G., and Sokolov, V., Immunomorphological studies on synthesis of melatonin in enterochromaffin cells, *Acta Histochem. Cytochem.,* 11, 75, 1978.

34. Grota, L.J. and Brown, G.M., Antibodies to indolealkylamines: serotonin and melatonin, *Can. J. Biochem.,* 52, 196, 1974.

35. Holloway, W.R., Grota, L.J., and Brown, G.M., Determination of imunoreactive melatonin in the colon of the rat by immunocytochemistry, *J. Histochem. Cytochem.,* 28, 255, 1980.

36. Quay, W.B. and Ma, Y.H., Demonstration of gastrointestinal hydroxyindole-*O*-methyltransferase, *IRCS Med. Sci.,* 4, 563, 1976.

37. Hong, G.X. and Pang, S.F., *N*-acetyltransferase activity in the quail (*Coturnix coturnix jap*) duodenum, *Comp. Biochem. Physiol.,* 112B, 251, 1995.

38. Reiter R.J., Pineal melatonin: cell biology of its synthesis and of its physiological interactions, *Endocrinol. Rev.*, 12, 151, 1991.

39. Pang S.F. and Allen A.E., Extrapineal melatonin in the retina: its regulation and physiological functions, *Pineal Res. Rev.*, 4, 55, 1986.

40. Bubenik, G.A., Localization of melatonin in the digestive tract of the rat. Effect of maturation, diurnal variation, melatonin treatment and pinealectomy, *Hormone Res.*, 12, 205, 1980.

41. Vakkuri, O., Rintamaki, H., and Leppaluoto, J., Presence of immunoreactive melatonin in different tissues of the pigeon (*Columbia livia*), *Gen. Comp. Endocrinol.*, 58, 69, 1985.

42. Illnerova, H., The effect of light on the development of hydroxyindole-*O*-methyltransferase activity in the rat pineal gland, *Acta Nervosa Super Praque*, 14, 130, 1972.

43. Bubenik, G.A. and Pang S.F., The role of serotonin and melatonin in the gastrointestinal physiology: ontogeny, regulation of food intake and mutual 5-HT melatonin feedbacks, *J. Pineal Res.*, 16, 91, 1994.

44. Bubenik, G.A., Phylogeny, ontogeny and function of gastrointestinal melatonin, presented at 5th Canadian Pineal and Melatonin Symposium, Guelph, July 13 to 15, 1997.

45. Bubenik, G.A., Niles, L.P., Pang, S.F., and Pentney, P.J., Diurnal variation and binding characteristics of melatonin in the mouse brain and gastrointestinal tissues, *Comp. Biochem. Physiol.*, 104C, 221, 1993.

46. Lee, P.N., Shiu, S.Y.W., Chow P.H., and Pang S.F., Regional and diurnal studies of melatonin and melatonin binding sites in the duck gastrointestinal tract, *Biol. Signals*, 4, 212, 1995.

47. Ozaki, Y. and Lynch, H.J., Presence of melatonin in plasma and urine of pinealectomized rats, *Endocrinoloy*, 99, 641, 1976.

48. Kennaway, D.J., Frith, K.G., Phillipou, G., Matthews, C.E., and Seamark, R.F., A specific radioimmunoassay for melatonin in biological tissue and fluids and its validation by gas-chromatography-mass spectrometry, *Endocrinology*, 110, 119, 1977.

49. Pang S.F., Woo, N.Y.S., Tang, P.L., and Allen A.E., Differential effect of bilateral enucleation on serum melatonin: evidence for an endocrine retina in fish and hypothesis of a sensori-hormonal transducer. *Chin. J. Physiol. Sci.*, 3, 341, 1987.

50. Kezuka, H. Iiogo, M. Furukawa, K. Aida, K., and Hanyu, I., Effects of photoperiod, pinealectomy and ophtalmectomy on circulating melatonin rhythms in the goldfish (*Carassius auratus*), *Zool. Sci.*, 9, 1047, 1992.

51. Huether, G, Hajak, G., Reimer, A., Poeggeler, R., Blomer, M., Rodenbeck, A., and Ruther E., The metabolic fate of infused L-tryptophan in men: possible clinical implications of the accumulation of circulating tryptophan and tryptophan metabolites, *Psychopharmacology*, 106, 422, 1992.

52. Huether, G., Poegeller, B., Reimer, R., and George A., Effect of tryptophan administration on circulating melatonin levels in chicks and rats: evidence for stimulation of melatonin synthesis and release in the gastrointestinal tract, *Life Sci.*, 51, 945, 1992.

53. Yaga, K., Reiter, R.J., and Richardson, B.A., Tryptophan loading increases daytime serum melatonin in intact and pinealectomized rats, *Life Sci.*, 52, 1231, 1993.

54. Krieger, D.T., Hauser, H., and Krey, L.C., Suprachiasmatic nuclear lesions do not abolish food-shifted circadian rhythmicity and temperature rhythmicity, *Science*, 197, 398, 1977.

55. Ho, A.K., Burns, T.G, Grota, L.J., and Brown, G.M., Scheduled feeding and 24-hour rhythms of *N*-acetylserotonin and melatonin in rats, *Endocrinology*, 116, 1858, 1985.

56. DeBoer, H., The Influence of Photoperiod and Melatonin on Hormone Levels, and Operand Light Demand in the Pig, Ph.D. thesis, University of Guelph, Ontario, Canada, 1988.

57. Rice, J., Mayor, J., Tucker, H.A., and Bielski R.J., Effect of light therapy on salivary melatonin in seasonal affective disorder, *Psychiatry Res.*, 56, 221, 1995.

58. Welker, H.A. and Vollrath, L., The effects of a number of short term exogenous stimuli on pineal serotonin-*N*-acetyltransferase activity in rats, *Cell Tiss. Res.*, 217, 105, 1984.

59. Chik, C.L., Ho, A.K., and Brown, G.M., Effect of food restriction on 24-hr serum and pineal melatonin content in male rat, *Acta Endocrinol.*, 115, 507, 1985.

60. Peacock, A.J., Thacher, P.A., Kirkwood R.N., and Tedesco, S., The effect of feed restriction and of beta-adrenergic agonist on plasma concentrations of melatonin in domestic pigs, *Can. J. Anim. Sci.*, 75, 203, 1995.

61. Breitins, I.Z., Barkan, A., Klibanski, A., Kyung, A.N., Reppert, S.M., Badger, T.M., Veldhuis, J.W., and McArthur, J.W., Hormonal responses to short-term fasting in postmenopausal women. *J. Clin. Endocrinol. Metab.*, 60, 1120, 1985.

62. Ferrari, E., Poppa, S., Bossolo, P.A., Comis, S., Esposti, G., Licini, V., Fraschini, F., and Brambila, F., Melatonin and pituitary-gonadal function in disorders of eating behavior, *J. Pineal Res.*, 7, 115, 1989.

63. Rojdmark, S. and Wetterberg, L., Short-term fasting inhibits the nocturnal melatonin secretion in healthy man, *Clin. Endocrinol.*, 30, 451, 1989.

64. Rojdmark, S., Rossner, S., and Wetterberg L., Effect of short-term fasting on nocturnal melatonin secretion in obesity, *Metabolism*, 41, 1106, 1992.

65. Benouali, S. Srada, N. Gharib, A., and Roche, M., Role of melatonin in the regulation of the interdigestive ileo-ceco-colic electromyogram in the rat, *C. R. Acad. Sci. Paris Life Sci.*, 316, 524, 1993 (in French).

66. Benouali-Pellissier, S., Melatonin is involved in cholecystokinin-induced changes of ileal motility in rats, *J. Pineal Res.*, 17, 79, 1994.

67. Kopin, I.J., Pare, C.M., Axelrod, J., and Weissbach, H., The fate of melatonin, *J. Biol. Chem.*, 236, 3072, 1961.

68. Petrova, G.A., Dedenkov, A.N., and Levin, I.M., Experimental and clinical study of diagnostic usefelness of melatonin determination in cancer patients, in Cyb, A.F. and Kvetnoy, I.M., Eds., *Regulatory Peptides and Biogenic Amines: Radiological and Oncological Aspects*, Russian Academy of Science, Obninsk, Russia, 1992, 58 (in Russian).

69. Pontoire, C., Bernard, M., Silvain, C., Collin, J.P., and Voisin, P., Characterization of melatonin biding sites in chicken and human intestines, *Eur. J. Pharmacol.*, 247, 111, 1993.

70. Poon, A.M.S., Mak, A.S., and Luk, H.T., Melatonin and [^{125}I]iodomelatonon binding sites in the human colon, *Endocrinol. Res.* 22, 77, 1991.

71. Cho, H.C., Pang, S.F., Chen, B.W., and Pfeifer, C.J., Modulating action of melatonin on serotonin-induced aggravation of ethanol ulceration and changes of mucosal blood flow in rat stomach, *J. Pineal Res.*, 6, 89, 1989.

72. Khan, R., Daya, S., and Potgieter, B., Evidence for the modulation of the stress response by the pineal gland, *Experientia*, 46, 860, 1990.

73. Ayles, H.L., Ball, R.O., Friendship, R.M., and Bubenik, G.A., The effect of graded levels of melatonin on performance and gastric ulcers in pigs, *Can. J. Anim. Sci.*, 76, 607, 1996.

74. Konturek, P.C., Konturek, S.J., Brzozowski, T., Dembinski, A., Zembala, M., Mytar, B., and Hahn, E.G., Gastroprotective activity of melatonin and its precursor, L-tryptophan, against stress-induced and ischemia-induced lesions is mediated by scavenge of oxygen radicals. *Scand. J. Gastroenterol.*, 32, 433, 1997.

75. Konturek, P.C., Konturek, S., Majka, J., Zembala, M., and Hahn, E.G., Melatonin affords protection against gastric lesions induced by ischemia-reperfusion possibly due to its antioxidant and mucosal microcirculatory effects, *Eur. J. Pharmacol.*, 122, 73, 1997.

76. Tache, Y., Stevens, R.L., and Ishikawa, T., Central nervous system action of TRH influences gastrointestinal function and ulceration, *Ann. N.Y. Acad. Sci.*, 553, 269, 1989.

77. Pentney, P. and Bubenik, G.A., Melatonin reduces the severity of dextran-induced colitis in mice, *J. Pin. Res.*, 19, 31, 1995.

78. Maestroni, J.M., The immunoneuroendocrine role of melatonin, *J. Pineal Res.*, 14, 1, 1993.

79. Poon, A.M.S. and Pang, S.F., Pineal melatonin-immune system interaction, *Frontiers in Hormone Research*, 21, 71, 1996.

80. Zerek-Melen, G., Lewinski, A., and Kulak, J., The opposite effect of high and low doses of melatonin upon mitotic activity of the mouse intestinal epithelium, *Endokrynol. Pol.*, 38, 317, 1987.

81. Legris, G.J., Will, P.C., and Hopfer, U., Inhibition of amiloride-sensitive sodium conductance by indolealkylamines, *Proc. Natl. Acad. Sci. USA*, 79, 2046, 1982.

82. Kvetnoy, I.M. and Levin, I.M., Diurnal melatonin excretion in gastric and rectal cancer patients, *Voprosy Onkologii*, 33, 29, 1987 (in Russian).

83. Vician, M., Zeman, M., Herichova, I., Jurani, M., Blazicek, P., and Matis, P., Melatonin content in plasma, saliva and large intestine of patients with colonic cancer, presented at 5th Canadian Pineal and Melatonin Symp., Guelph, July 13 to 15, 1997.

84. Pentney, P., An Investigation of Melatonin in the Gastrointestinal Tract, M.Sc. thesis, University of Guelph, Ontario, Canada, 1995.

85. Weissbluth, L. and Weissbluth, M., Infant colic: the effect of serotonin and melatonin circadian rhythms on the intestinal smooth muscle, *Med. Hypotheses,* 39, 164, 1992.

86. Brown, G.M., Grota, L.J., Bubenik, G.A., Niles, S., and Tsui, H., Physiological regulation of melatonin, *Adv. Biosci.,* 29, 95, 1980.

Chapter **3**

The Antioxidant Properties of Melatonin

David Solkoff, William T. Cummings, Bailin Liang,
Paula Inserra, and Ronald R. Watson

Contents

Introduction

In 1959, the chemical structure of the indoleamine melatonin (*N*-acetyl-5-methoxytryptamine) was determined following its isolation from mammalian pineal glands.[1] The production of melatonin is modulated by the photoperiodic environment. In all vertebrates studied, melatonin is made and secreted in a circadian rhythm, with normal synthesis and release being minimized in periods of daylight and maximized during darkness.[2] Thus, the pineal hormone has been connected to the control of 24-hr cycles through its action on a reputed biological clock, the suprachiasmatic nuclei (SCN).[3]

Melatonin is easily and quickly taken up by cells because it is very lipid soluble and fairly water soluble. It has also been shown to cross physiological barriers readily, including the blood-brain barrier. Therefore, melatonin is believed to be accessible to all cells.[4,5]

The actions of melatonin are believed to be mediated through receptors on cell membranes. Membrane receptors for this hormone have been described in various areas within the brain including the SCN.[6,7] A membrane receptor for melatonin has been cloned and determined to be a member of the G-protein-linked receptor super-family.[8,9] Membrane receptors for melatonin have also been shown to exist on immune cells, and most of these membrane receptors use cyclic AMP (cAMP) as their intracellular second messenger.[10]

Besides having receptors for melatonin on cell membranes, investigative studies have found nuclear binding sites for this indoleamine. First shown in hepatic cell nuclei, these receptors have been determined to exist within the nuclei of cells present in the central nervous system and peripheral structures.[11-14] In addition to its receptor mediated effects, melatonin has receptor-independent actions. For example, because it can readily diffuse across cell membranes, it has been shown to bind and antago-nize calmodulin inside the cell, thus influencing calcium-dependent intracellular events, such as the inhibition of Ca^{2+}/calmodulin-dependent cerebellar nitric oxide synthase (NOS) activity.[15-18]

Melatonin has been promoted as a treatment for "jet lag" and insomnia.[19,20] In addition to being touted as having life-prolonging, anti-aging properties,[21,22] it has been shown to modulate various physiological systems.[23,24] The hormone has been connected to the neuroendocrine system, through its ability to control reproductive physiology in photoperiodic rodents.[25] With the passing of time, the interrelationship between the pineal gland, melatonin, seasonally changing photoperiods, and annual variations in reproductive capabilities has become better understood. This increased knowledge was the basis for studying melatonin as a human contraceptive agent, particularly because it would be free of the negative side-effects associated with estrogen-based contraceptives.[26,27] The pineal hormone has also been determined to exercise a significant influence on the proper functioning of the immune system.[28]

In spite of the fact that oxygen is required for aerobic organisms to live, once metabolized, oxygen can be potentially harmful. The majority of the O_2 (molecular oxygen, dioxygen) that is drawn into an organism's body is used to produce energy in the form of adenosine triphosphate (ATP); however, up to 5% of the O_2 in an organism is converted to reactive oxygen species (ROS) or free radicals.[29] Free radicals are molecules or parts of molecules which have one or more unpaired electrons. They often have an independent, yet very short-lived existence. Electrons are electrically charged and usually paired. While rotating, they induce a magnetic field or spin. An electron doublet is more stable than two isolated electrons, as the pairing of two electrons with opposite spin cancels their reciprocal magnetic fields. A free radical, by contrast, is a neutral or charged chemical species whose outer shell contains an unpaired electron, thus possessing an odd amount of electrons.[30,31] This lone electron gives a species such as the hydroxyl radical instability in terms of energy and kinetics. Energetically, in order to achieve a level of stability, free radicals seek to eliminate lone electrons from their electron inventory. This may be done either by losing an electron, thereby making the radical a reducing species (as with COO') or by gaining an electron, which would classify the radical as an oxidizing species such as OH'.[32] It should be noted that through a dismutation reaction a radical can often self-oxidize; consider the reaction in Equation 1:

$$O_2^{\cdot} + O_2^{\cdot} \xrightarrow{2H^+} H_2O_2 + O_2 \qquad \text{(Eq. 1)}$$

In this reaction (demonstrated *in vitro*), one of the two radicals is oxidizing while the other is reducing. *In vivo*, this reaction is catalyzed by one of several isoforms of an enzyme known as superoxide dismutase (SOD). As shown above, hydrogen peroxide may form as a result of the superoxide anion's dismutation reaction; however, it may also be produced from a bivalent reduction of O_2. The addition of the second electron leads to the formation of hydrogen peroxide, which is a powerful oxidizing agent.[32] Due to the unpaired electrons in their outer shells, free radicals are favored to pair with other molecules during bimolecular collisions. Because these types of collisions occur so frequently, these reactions are known to be very rapid, as the rate is determined by the efficiency of collisions.[32]

The term ROS is used to classify the products of O_2 which do not contribute to the synthesis of ATP. They include oxygen free radicals such as superoxide anion ($O_2^{\cdot}$), hydroxyl radical ('OH), peroxyl radical ($RO_2^{\cdot}$), and alkoxyl radical (RO').[33] Non-free radicals that may be classified as ROS include hydrogen peroxide (H_2O_2), hypochlorous acid (HOCl), singlet oxygen ($^1O_2$), and ozone (O_3). The superoxide anion is produced by the monovalent reduction of molecular oxygen. This occurs when O_2 picks up one lone electron with its accompanying supply of energy. *In vivo*, $O_2^{\cdot}$ may cause damage indirectly, as superoxide anion is a precursor of the highly toxic hydroxyl radical. This results from the Haber and Weiss reaction (Equation 2):

$$O_2^{\cdot} + H_2O_2 \rightarrow O_2 + OH^- + OH^{\cdot} \qquad \text{(Eq. 2)}$$

In another example of free radical formation known as the Fenton process, H_2O_2, in the presence of ferrous ions (Fe^{2+}), decomposes into a harmless OH^- ion and a powerful OH' radical. OH' has the ability to attack stable organic structures (Equation 3). This slow reaction process requires the presence of ferric ions which act as a catalyst.

$$O_2^{\cdot} + Fe^{3+} \rightarrow O_2 + Fe^{2+}$$
$$Fe^{2+} + H_2O_2 \rightarrow Fe^{3+} + OH^- + OH^{\cdot} \qquad \text{(Eq. 3)}$$

The reactivity of hydroxyl radicals is high in biological media, and their reactions with neighboring molecules results in the production of secondary radicals, either by the loss of a hydrogen atom or by transfer of the lone electron. Alkoxy radicals and peroxy radicals are produced from polyunsaturated fatty acid (PUFA) chains through the actions of oxygen free radicals, such as superoxide anions or hydroxyl radicals. Peroxy radicals are known to be more selective and less reactive than hydroxyl radicals. They are responsible for chain reactions such as the basic process for lipid peroxidation in cell membranes.

Even though free radicals are a type of ROS and thus a part of the underlying basis for many diseases, they also carry out some necessary and beneficial functions.[34–36] Certain ROS are required for the phagocytic functions of cells, and may sometimes function as intracellular signaling molecules.[36–39] In certain instances, the *in vivo* production of oxygen free radicals may be regarded as "inadvertent". These may include such occurrences as the synthesis of superoxide anions following the leakage of electrons from the electron transport chain and the production of hydroxyl radical by the cleavage of water when organisms are exposed to background ionizing radiation. Levels of free radicals can also be increased during exposure to ultraviolet (UV) light or in the metabolism of antibiotics.[33]

Free radicals are formed *in vivo* primarily because the oxygen molecule undergoes enzymatic reductions which are involved in electron transport. These include certain processes in the mitochondrial respiratory chain, the actions of oxygenase group enzymes, oxygen binding to hemoglobin, and interactions of oxygen with auto-oxidizable molecules such as catecholamines, riboflavin, melanins, or glycoproteins. Oxidative reactions during detoxification also produce free radicals by the actions of oxidases contained in peroxysomes. Cytochrome P450 is a complex of proteins that also produce free radicals via their function as oxidases through single electron transfers.[32] Free radicals can also originate in an exogenous fashion, being formed by X-ray and gamma-ray ionizing radiation. As its energy levels lessen in strength, the radiation withdraws an electron from certain molecules in its path, causing the radiolysis of water present in the exposed tissues.[40]

The Potential of Free Radicals To Cause Harm

DNA Damage

Free radicals such as OH˙ damage subcellular components. This damage accumulates as an organism ages and may, in part, account for aging and age-related diseases.[41,42] The hydroxyl radical has been shown to increase the likelihood of developing cancer, as it is toxic enough to damage DNA.[43] It is known to attack the sugars of bases in such a way as to produce strand breaks, cause base modifications, and create lesions that may result in mutations and cancer.[44] The molecular devastation caused by free radical attack is known as oxidative damage, while the nonstop assault on molecules by ROS (as many as 10,000 strikes against the DNA of each cell each day) is called oxidative stress.[25,45] Even though DNA repair enzymes remove many of the lesions, some damage always remains, as the repair processes are not 100% effective.[46] Evidence of this damage has been described in studies that show about one million DNA lesions per cell in a 3-month-old rat, while a 24-month-old rat had about 2 million per cell. Additionally, a 900% increase in lymphocyte mutation frequency among elderly human subjects as compared to newborns has been described.[47] Since mitochondrial DNA (mtDNA) is located near the superoxide anions leaking from the electron transport chain, mtDNA is particularly subjected to oxidative attack. Oxidative lesions in the mtDNA of liver cells have been observed to occur as much as nine times more frequently as they do in nuclear DNA, so they are always producing new mitochondria to compensate for this high degree of damage. In spite of this protection strategy, damaged mtDNA accumulates quicker than damaged nuclear DNA.[48]

Damage to Proteins

Proteins are highly vulnerable to oxidative attack because of their large size and because some tend to associate with transition metals, such as iron.[49] Tyrosine, phenylalanine, tryptophan, histadine, methionine, and cysteine residues are the preferred targets, even though all amino acid residues can be damaged by free radicals.[50] Changes in the fluorescent properties of protein molecules occur as amino acid residues are oxidized because of the resulting physical/conformational modifications that the protein undergoes. These physical changes are usually of three types: fragmentations, aggregations, or changes rendering the protein susceptible to proteolytic digestion.[51-52] Examples of proteins studied with respect to oxidative damage are collagen and albumin, both of which experience fragmentation when oxidized by free radicals. Two proteins found to undergo denaturation and aggregation when attacked by free radicals are Cu-binding ceruloplasmin and lenticular protein.[33] The process of aggregation has been attributed to the ability of hydroxyl radicals to form cross-linkages.[53] When a protein becomes denatured by interacting with free radicals and undergoes a conformational change, it is likely to be enzymatically degraded, resulting in a decrease in the metabolic efficiency of cells. Therefore, it is likely that oxidation of proteins is increased when oxygen free radical production is elevated.

Damage to Lipids

Free radical production results in additional cellular damage because they cause peroxidation of lipids. Lipid peroxidation damages cell membranes. The membrane loses fluidity and has decreased electrical resistance. Membrane protein mobility is decreased, and there can be an increase in the phospholipid exchange between the bilayers of the membrane.[54] If unchecked, cell membrane damage can be so severe as to cause inactivation of membrane-bound enzymes and an overall compromise in the structural integrity of the cell.

Although the specific mechanisms by which lipids undergo peroxidation were learned mainly from *in vitro* studies, the process is thought to occur also *in vivo*.

Furthermore, biologically active aldehydes are produced as intermediates in the lipid peroxidation process. One example is malonaldehyde which can cross-link and aggregate membrane proteins. When the sum total is considered, aldehydes, free radicals, and other products of lipid peroxidation can cause destruction of membrane proteins.[33] Consider the peroxidation of PUFA. It has been shown to happen in three stages: initiation, propagation, and termination.[55] Initiation starts with the removal of hydrogen atoms from the lipid molecule which results in the formation of carbon-centered free radicals that contain conjugated diene bonds. This can be caused by a variety of initiating radicals.[56] Redox-active metals, such as iron and copper, have been found to assist in this process.[57] In the propagation phase of lipid peroxidation, oxygen reacts with the carbon-centered free radicals, resulting in the formation of peroxyl radicals. These peroxyl radicals can then react with another PUFA, thus propagating the chain reaction and forming lipid peroxides (also called lipid hydro-peroxides). It has been demonstrated *in vitro* that until it is stopped, this chain reaction has the potential to damage all accessible PUFA.[58] This reaction can there-fore be considered substrate limited. It should be noted, however, that radical-radical interactions do occur that result in the termination of the chain reaction that causes the formation of lipid peroxides. It has been shown that if two lipid radicals unite, nonradical products will be formed.[59] The same chain termination occurs when a lipid radical interacts with a peroxyl radical.

Protection Against Free Radicals

The Antioxidant Defense Repertoire

There are several endogenous and exogenous compounds that offer antioxidant protection against free radicals (see Table 1). Notwithstanding the action of the antioxidant substances listed in the table, molecules suffer free radical oxidant damage. This damage may be responsible, at least in part, for aging and age-related diseases.[42,53,60-63] This damage can be caused by environmental insults such as ultraviolet radiation. It may also result from physical stress such as excessive exer-cise, psychological stress, or exposure to toxins.

Melatonin as an Antioxidant

In 1993, *in vitro* evidence was reported that melatonin was a voracious scavenger or inhibitor of the very toxic hydroxyl radical.[64] It was thought that melatonin might modulate the redox state of cells, as it could promote Ca^{2+}-stimulated and Mg^{2+}-dependent ATPase (calcium pump) activity in cardiac muscle tissue (even though this tissue was apparently lacking melatonin receptors).[65] To test the ability of the hormone to modulate the redox state of cells, an *in vitro* experimental model was devised in order to determine melatonin's ability to neutralize OH.

TABLE 1
Oxygen-Based Free Radicals and the Antioxidants
That Either Metabolize or Scavenge Them

Free Radical	Antioxidant
Singlet oxygen	α-Tocopherol, β-carotene, bilirubin, cholesterol, histidine, reduced glutathione, reduced PUFA
Hydrogen peroxide	Catalase, glutathione peroxidase
Superoxide anion	Vitamin C (ascorbate), tyrosamine, reduced glutathione, superoxide dismutases
Hydroxyl radical	Vitamin C, uric acid, reduced PUFA, methionine, melatonin, mannitol, DNA bases (guanine, cytosine, uracil), butanol ethanol, benzoate

Note: The enzymes listed on this table metabolize the radicals to other compounds. The remaining antioxidants listed scavenge them.

A solution of H_2O_2 was exposed to 254-nm ultraviolet light to generate a hydroxyl radical:

$$H_2O_2 \xrightarrow[\text{UV light}]{254\ nm} OH^{\bullet} + OH^{\bullet} \qquad \textbf{(Eq. 4)}$$

A major problem to be overcome was determining the quantity of OH· present at a given point in time. This problem arises because the half-life of OH· is very brief (approximately 10^{-9} sec).[66] In order to resolve this impediment, a radical spin-trapping agent was added to the H_2O_2 solution. The chosen spin trap was 5,5-dimethyl pyroline-*N*-oxide (DMPO). This chemical forms fairly stable adducts with OH·. Therefore, the adducts can be used to discern indirectly the amount of OH· in solution:

$$H_2O_2 + DMPO \xrightarrow[\text{UV light}]{254\ nm} DMPO - OH^{\bullet} \qquad \textbf{(Eq. 5)}$$

High-performance liquid chromatography (HPLC) with electrochemical detection, in addition to electron spin resonance spectroscopy, was conducted to identify and quantify the adducts.[67] Melatonin and other known radical scavengers such as glutathione and mannitol were then added to determine the effectiveness of melatonin's ability to neutralize the hydroxyl radical. Results showed melatonin to be the best of the three at this task. The pharmacological concentration of melatonin necessary to scavenge 50% of the radicals produced (IC_{50}) was 21 μM; by contrast, the IC_{50} for glutathione was 123 μM, and for mannitol was 283 μM.[64] Remarkably, melatonin was five times better at scavenging than glutathione and 15 times better than mannitol. In the same study, naturally occurring analogs of melatonin were reported to be less effective, or totally ineffective, as free radical scavengers. When tested in other *in vitro* systems, including one utilizing [2,2'-azio-*bis*-3-ethylbenz-thiazoline-

6-sulfonic acid] (ABTS+ cation radical), it performed in a similar manner.[68,69] *In vitro,* melatonin has been shown to work even better when it combines its activity synergistically with vitamin C, Trolox (liquid vitamin E), and glutathione to reduce the formation of the ABTS+ cation radical. This synergistic relationship is believed to occur *in vivo,* as well.[70]

A free radical scavenger will come to possess an unpaired electron once it has contributed an electron to neutralize a free radical. Paradoxically, the free radical scavenger becomes a free radical! When melatonin neutralizes the toxic ˙OH it becomes an indolyl cation radical. However, this molecule has been shown to have low toxicity.[68,71] This radical then has the capability to scavenge a superoxide anion and in the process is converted to N^1-acetyl-N^2-formyl-5-methoxykynuramine (AMFK). In this way, melatonin utilizes a second mechanism to neutralize ˙OH, as superoxide anion is a precursor of much of the ˙OH generated *in vivo.*[71]

Further experiments tested the ability of melatonin to scavenge the peroxyl radical. Because vitamin E is a known effective neutralizer of peroxyl radicals, melatonin's effectiveness was compared against that of Trolox.[72] Using an *in vitro* model, it was reported that melatonin was approximately twice as effective as Trolox at scavenging the peroxyl radical. In all *in vitro* studies conducted thus far, melatonin has shown itself to be the most effective warrior against free radicals.

With respect to *in vivo* studies investigating the antioxidant potential of melatonin, the hormone has been found to provide antioxidant protection to an array of macromolecules, including DNA, proteins, and lipids. The antioxidant protective actions of melatonin have been demonstrated in the membranes, cytosol, and nuclei of cells.

Melatonin Protects DNA

In vivo, the chemical carcinogen safrole causes DNA damage by inducing nuclear toxic free radicals, especially in liver cells.[73] In order to see if melatonin could protect liver cell DNA from free radical damage, rats were treated with safrole (300 mg/kg) with and without simultaneous melatonin administration (either 0.2 or 0.4 mg/kg). Twenty four hours later, the livers of each animal was harvested, and total hepatic DNA was isolated and postlabeled with ^{32}P.[74] DNA adducts were separated by chromatography, and autoradiograms were prepared and were quantified using a Beta Scope. Melatonin provided hepatic DNA with a high degree of protection from free radical damage instigated by safrole. A dose of melatonin that was 1500 times less than the administered dose of safrole was sufficient to reduce DNA damage by approximately 40%.[75] When the administered dose of melatonin was doubled, production of DNA adducts was only about 5% higher than controls.

In an effort to test the antioxidant properties of melatonin against the potent ˙OH, ionizing radiation was administered to human lymphocytes with or without melatonin. Ionizing radiation was chosen, as it is known to cause the formation of oxygen-based radicals which can damage genetic material.[76,77] As a positive control, a known free radical scavenger (dimethyl sulfoxide, DMSO) was incubated with some of the cell samples. After incubating the lymphocytes with the above-mentioned compounds, they were irradiated with a total dose of 150 cGY/min. After 48 hr, the cells were analyzed cytogenetically for chromosomal damage. Exchange aberrations, acentric fragments, and micronuclei were counted as damage. With respect to all parameters, melatonin reduced damage in a dose-dependent manner. At 2.0 mM, ionizing radiation damage to chromosomes was reduced by approximately 70%. In order for DMSO to show that kind of result, a concentration 500 times greater than that of melatonin had to be used.[76–80] Further experiments have shown that mice have a better chance of surviving ionizing radiation pretreated with melatonin.[80] Due to its powerful antioxidative potential, it has been postulated that melatonin helps to preserve the overall integrity of DNA and in so doing reduces the liklihood of cancer.

Melatonin Protects Proteins

There is evidence suggesting that melatonin offers antioxidant protection to proteins, particularly from a study involving cataract formation in newborn rats. Cataracts are known to arise from the oxidation of proteins in the lens by oxygen-based radicals; therefore, an experiment was conducted in order to test the ability of melatonin to prevent cataract formation. Shortly after birth, newborn rats were treated with buthionine sulfoximine (BSO), which is an inhibitor of glutathione synthesis. Without glutathione, rats suffer increased oxidative damage to lenticular protein, resulting in cataracts by 2 weeks of age. These rats are also deficient in melatonin, as it is only minimally produced during the rat pup's first half-month of life. The study showed that melatonin was able to prevent cataract development almost totally when given to these glutathione-deficient rats during the first 2 weeks of life. Because melatonin levels drop significantly in advanced old age, replacement therapy may help to alleviate senile cataracts, a major problem associated with aging.[81–85]

Protection of Lipids by Melatonin

The first studies to show that melatonin decreases the peroxidation of lipids did not indicate that it was very potent in this regard. It was found that melatonin pretreatment limited the rise in blood glucose that normally follows the administration of alloxan to mice. Alloxan is known to destroy the insulin-secreting β-cells of the pancreas through free-radical mechanisms. It was also found that melatonin (and to a greater degree 6-hydroxymelatonin) reduced the production of lipid peroxides in mouse brain homogenates induced by thiobarbituric reactive substances.[86] Accordingly, it has been suggested that part of the antioxidative ability of melatonin *in vivo* may be due to its conversion to the above-mentioned hepatic metabolite. Later studies used paraquat, a highly toxic xenobiotic, to induce the destruction of lipids in rat lungs. Paraquat administration caused extensive lipid peroxidation as indicated by increased levels of malondialdehyde (MDA) and 4-hydroxyalkenals (4-HDA) in the lungs. Concomitant with this increase in MDA and 4-HDA levels, there was a significant decrease in glutathione concentrations, another indication of severe oxidative stress. Melatonin administration given in conjunction with paraquat comprehensively inhibited the above-stated oxidative changes. When the animals were given melatonin (10 mg/kg) the paraquat LD_{50} rose from 80 mg/kg to approximately 250 mg/kg within 24 hr.[87] In another experiment, melatonin administration was found to be similarly effective in inhibiting MDA and 4-HDA accumulation in various rat tissues, when these tissues were challenged with bacterial lipopolysaccharide (LPS). LPS is a potent endotoxin known to cause multiple organ damage by free radical mechanisms.[88] In a further study, mice were fed dextran sodium sulfate (DSS) in order to induce colitis. DSS promotes the proliferation of gram-negative bacteria in the gastrointestinal tract, resulting in excessive production of LPS endotoxin. When the mice were given melatonin in addition to DSS, the severity of the colitis symptoms was significantly reduced, presumably due to the ability of the pineal indole to neutralize the various free radicals produced under these conditions.[89-91] In another demonstration of the ability of melatonin to reduce (in a dose-dependent manner) the level of lipid peroxidation products, liver homogenates or microsomes were incubated with either carbon tetrachloride (CCl_4, a widely used solvent and cleaning chemical) or CCl_4 plus melatonin. When ingested, CCl_4 severely damages liver tissue, and this damage is considered to be free-radical based. When melatonin was administered, however, beneficial results similar to those previously described above were obtained against CCl_4.[92-94]

Lipid peroxidation is also known to occur when retina or brain tissue homogenates are incubated with both H_2O_2 and $FeSO_4$. This rise in lipid peroxidation products was found to be markedly inhibited when pharmacological doses of melatonin were added to the incubation media.[95-97] Another study showing that melatonin, *in vitro*, reduces oxidative damage to lipids found that the hormone, in a dose-dependent manner, diminished the accumulation of some of the major products of lipid peroxidation, namely MDA and 4-HDA. In this study, rat brain homogenates were treated with kainic acid, a highly neurotoxic, nondegradable analog of the excitatory neurotransmitter glutamate. When injected into animals, kainic acid causes seizures and neuronal damage. Marked lipid peroxidation was observed when rat brain homogenates of striatum, hypothalamus, hippocampus, cerebellum, and cerebral cortex, were incubated with 11.7 mM kainic acid. In homogenates that were coincubated with melatonin (0.1 to 0.4 mM), lipid peroxidation was suppressed. In some cases, the highest concentrations of melatonin were able to reduce MDA and 4-HDA levels in homogenates treated with kainic acid to levels below those seen in control mice not incubated with kainic acid, thus indicating decreased lipid peroxidation.[98] The study discussed above and other studies suggest that melatonin protects the brain from kainic acid due to its direct free-radical scavenging capability.[99]

Other Evidence of Antioxidative Properties of Melatonin

At the molecular level, melatonin has been shown to inhibit the activation of the transcriptional regulator nuclear factor NF-κB, whose activation involves free radicals as second messengers. NF-κB binding to DNA was stimulated by exposing HeLa S3 cells to tumor necrosis factor-α, phorbol-12-myristate-13-acetate, or ionizing radiation, all of which generate intracellular free radicals. When melatonin was added at concentrations as low as 10 μM, the activation of NF-κB was inhibited by each of the aforementioned agents. This inhibition is believed, once again, to be due to the ability of melatonin to neutralize free radicals.[100]

Melatonin has been shown to stimulate the activity of glutathione peroxidase, an important antioxidative enzyme in the brain. By doing this, it would promote the metabolism of hydrogen peroxide and lipid peroxides, thus reducing the damage caused by free radicals.[101] Furthermore, melatonin has recently been shown to be an effective scavenger of peroxynitrite, an ROS formed from nitric oxide and superoxide anion. The cytotoxic damage caused by peroxynitrite includes lipid peroxidation, a diminishing of mitochondrial respiration, depletion of glutathione, inhibition of membrane pumps, and damage to DNA with subsequent activation of poly (ADP ribose) synthetase and associated cellular energy depletion.[102–105]

Further evidence of the antioxidant powers of melatonin includes a recent study showing that exogeneously administered melatonin given to male rats protects against liver oxidative damage induced by the type of ischemic reperfusion injury known to be associated with liver trasnsplantation procedures. Results indicate reduced lipid peroxidation products, a reduction of the polymorphonuclear neutrophil infiltration that is known to occur in ischemic-reperfusion damaged livers, and increased glutathione levels.[104]

Conclusion

The recent accumulation of data clearly indicates that melatonin can exhibit potent antioxidant properties, significantly benefiting the defensive systems of organisms. Because melatonin has no known toxicity and is readily absorbed regardless of the route of administration, the findings described herein have important implications, even if the protective effects of melatonin can be achieved only at pharmacological rather than physiological doses. Previous studies have been able to approximate physiological doses of the hormone at 80 pg/ml at 25 years of age, 40 pg/ml at 55 years of age, and 25 pg/ml at 85 years of age.[62]

A question presently generating intense interest both academically and publicly is that, because free radicals play a role in promoting neurodegenerative diseases that increase with aging and because melatonin levels decrease with aging, can melatonin supplementation at least partially forestall age-related degenerative disease processes?

Acknowledgments

This review was stimulated by research supported by grants from Phi Beta Psi and the Wallace Genetics Foundation, Inc. Support was also obtained from The

University of Arizona College of Medicine Summertime Institute on Medical Igno-
rance and by The University of Arizona Department of Molecular and Cellular
Biology Undergraduate Biology Research Program, which is funded in part by The
National Science Foundation and The Howard Hughes Medical Institute.

References

1. Lerner, A.B., Case, J.B., and Heinzelman, R.V., Structure of melatonin, *J. Am. Chem. Soc.*, 81, 6084–6085, 1959.

2. Reiter, R.J.R., Pineal melatonin: cell biology of its synthesis and of its physiological interactions, *Endocrinol. Rev.*, 12, 151–180, 1991.

3. Cassone, V.M., Chesworth, M.J., and Armstrong, S., Entrainment of rat circadian rhythms by daily injection with melatonin depends upon the hypothalamic suprachiasmatic nucleus, *Physiol. Behav.*, 36, 111–121, 1986.

4. Shida, C.S., Castrucci, A.M., and Lamy-Freund, M.T., High melatonin solubility in aqueous medium, *J. Pineal Res.*, 16, 198–201, 1994.

5. Menendez-Palaez, A. and Reiter, R.J.R., The distribution of melatonin in mammalian tissues: the relative importance of nuclear versus cytosolic localization, *J. Pineal Res.*, 15, 59–69, 1993.

6. Morgan, J.P., Molecular signalling via the melatonin receptor, *Adv. Pineal Res.*, 5, 191–198, 1991.

7. Reppert, S.M., Weaver, D.R., Rivkees, S.A., and Stopa, E.G., Putative melatonin receptors in a human biological clock, *Science*, 242, 78–81, 1988

8. Ebisawa, T., Karne, S., Lerner, M.R., and Reppert, S.M., Expression cloning of high affinity melatonin receptor from *Xenopus* dermal melanophores, *Proc. Natl. Acad. Sci. USA*, 91, 6133–6137, 1994.

9. Reppert, S.M., Weaver, D.R., and Ebisawa, T., Cloning and characterization of a mammalian melatonin receptor that mediates reproductive and circadian responses, *Neuron*, 13, 1177–1185, 1994.

10. Poon, A.M. and Pang, S.F., Modulation of two [^{125}I]iodomelatonin binding sites in the guinea pig spleen by melatonin injection is dependent is dependent on the dose and period but not the time, *Life Sci.*, 54, 1411–1418, 1994.

11. Acuna-Castroviejo, D., Pablos, M.I., Menendez-Palaez, A., Reiter, R.J.R., Melatonin receptors in purified cell nuclei of liver, *Res. Commun. Chem. Pathol. Pharmacol.*, 82, 253–256, 1993.

12. Acuna-Castroviejo, D., Reiter, R.J.G., Menendez-Palaez, A., Pablos, M.I., Burgos, A., Characterization of high-affinity binding sites in purified cell nuclei of rat liver, *J. Pineal Res.*, 16,100–113, 1994.

13. Becker-Andre, M., Wiesenberg, I., Schaeren-Wiemers, N., Andre, E., Missbach, M., and Souret, J.H., Pineal hormone melatonin binds to and activates an orphan of the nuclear receptor superfamily, *J. Biol. Chem.*, 269, 28531–28534, 1994.

14. Carlberg, C. and Wiesenberg, I., The orphan receptor family RZR/ROR, melatonin, and 5-lipoxygenase: an unexpected relationship, *J. Pineal Res.,* 18, 171–178, 1995.

15. Huerto-Delgadillo, L., Anton-Tay, F., and Benitz-King, G., Effects of melatonin on microtubule assembly depend on hormone concentration: role of melatonin as a calmodulin antagonist, *J. Pineal Res.,* 13, 55–62, 1992.

16. Pozo, D., Reiter, R.J.R., Calvo, J.M., and Guerrero, J.M., Physiological concentrations of melatonin inhibit nitric oxide synthase in rat cerebellum, *Life Sci.,* 55, PL455–PL460, 1994.

17. Benitez-King, G., Huerto-Delgadillo, L., and Anton-Tay, F., Binding of ^{3}H-melatonin to calmodulin, *Life Sci.,* 53, 201–207, 1993.

18. Anton-Tay, F., Huerto-Delgadillo, L., Ortega-Corona, B., and Benitez-King, G., Melatonin antagonism to calmodulin may modulate multiple cellular functions, in Touitou, Y., Arendt, J., and Pevet, P., Eds., *Melatonin and the Pineal Gland: From Basic Science to Clinical Applications,* Excerpta Medica, Amsterdam, 1993, 41.

19. Arendt, J., Aldhous, M., English, J., and Marks, V., The effects of jet-lag and their alleviation by melatonin, *Ergonomics,* 30, 1379–1393, 1987.

20. Dawson, D. and Encel, N., Melatonin and sleep in humans, *J. Pineal Res.,* 15, 1–15, 1993.

21. Reiter, R.J.R., The aging pineal gland and its physiological consequences, *Bioessays,* 14, 169–175, 1992.

22. Pierpaoli, W. and Regelson, W., Pineal control of aging: effects of melatonin on aging mice, *Proc. Nat. Acad. Sci. USA,* 91, 787–791, 1994.

23. Cassone, V.M., Effects of melatonin on vertebrate circadian systems, *Trends Neurosci.,* 13, 457–464, 1990.

24. Blask, D.E., Melatonin in oncology, in Yu, H.S. and Reiter, R.J.R., Eds., *Melatonin,* CRC Press, Boca Raton, FL, 1993, 447–476, 1993.

25. Hoffman, R.A. and Reiter, R.J.R., Pineal gland: influence on gonads of male hamsters, *Science,* 148, 1609–1611, 1965.

26. Reiter, R.J.R., Comparative physiology: pineal gland, *Ann. Rev. Physiol.,* 35, 305–328, 1973.

27. Voordouw, B.C., Euser, R., Verdonk, R.E., Aberda, B.T., de Jong, F.H., and Drogendijk, A.C., Melatonin and melatonin progestin combinations alter pituitary-ovarian function in women and can inhibit ovulation, *J. Clin. Endocrinol. Metab.,* 74, 108–117, 1992.

28. Curoleo, M.C., Frasca, D., Nistico, G., and Doria, G., Melatonin as immunomodulator in immunodeficient mice, *Immunopharmacology,* 23, 81–89, 1992.

29. Floyd, R.A., Role of oxygen free radicals in carcinogenesis and brain ischemia, *FASEB J.,* 4, 2587–2597, 1990.

30. Buechter, D.D., Free radicals and oxygen toxicity, *Pharm. Res.,* 5, 253–260, 1988.

31. Halliwell, B., Free radicals and antioxidant protection mechanisms and significance in toxicology and disease, *Human Toxicol.,* 7, 7–13, 1988.

32. Pierrefiche, G. and Laborit, H., Oxygen free radicals, melatonin, and aging, *Exp. Gerontol.,* 30, 3–4, 213–227, 1995.

33. Reiter, R.J.R., The role of the neurohormone melatonin as a buffer against macromolecular oxidative damage, *Neurochem. Int.,* 6, 453–460, 1995.

34. Knight, J.A., Diseases related to oxygen derived free radicals, *Ann. Clin. Lab. Med.,* 25, 111–121, 1995.

35. Reiter, R.J.R., Oxidative processes and antioxidative defense mechanisms in the aging brain, *FASEB J.,* 9, 526–533, 1995.

36. Schreck, P. and Baurerle, P.A., A role of oxygen radicals as second messengers, *Trends Cell.Biol.,* 1, 39–42, 1991.

37. Root, R.K. and Metcalf, J.A., Hydrogen peroxide release from human granulocytes during phagocytosis, *J. Clin. Invest.,* 6, 1266–1279, 1977.

38. Babior, B.M., Oxygen dependent microbial killing by phagocytes, *N. Engl. J. Med.,* 298, 721–725, 1978.

39. Schreck, R., Rieber, P., and Bauererle, P.A., Reactive oxygen intermediates as apparently widely used messengers in the activation of the NF-κB transcription factor and HIV-1, *EMBO J.,* 10, 2247–2258, 1991.

40. Laborit, H., *Les Regulations Metaboliques,* Masson, Paris, 1965.

41. Harman, D., Free radical involvement in aging, *Drugs Aging,* 3, 60-80, 1993.

42. Harman, D., Aging: prospects for further increases in the functional life span, *Age,* 17, 119–146, 1994 .

43. Steenken, S., Purine bases, nucleosides, and nucleotides: aqueous solution redox chemistry and transformation reactions of their radical cations and OH adducts, *Chem. Rev.,* 89, 503–520, 1989.

44. Meneghini, R. and Martins, E.L., Hydrogen peroxide and DNA damage, in Halliwell, B. and Aruoma, O.I., Eds., *DNA and Free Radicals,* Harwood, London, 83–93, 1993.

45. Sies, H., Oxidative stress, in Sies, H., Ed., *Oxidative Stress,* Academic Press, New York, 1991, xv–xvii.

46. Ramotar, D. and Demple, B., Enzymes that repair oxidative damage to DNA, in Haliwell, B. and Aruoma, O.I., Eds., *DNA and Free Radicals,* Harwood, London, 165–192, 1993.

47. Ames, B.N. and Shigenaga, M.K., Oxidants are a major contributor to cancer and aging, in Halliwell, B. and Aruoma, O.I., Eds., *DNA and Free Radicals,* Harwood, London, 1–15, 1993.

48. Shigenaga, M.K. and Ames, B.N., Oxidants and mitochondrial decay in aging, in Frei, B., Ed., *Natural Antioxidants in Human Health and Disease,* Academic Press, San Diego, 63–106, 1994.

49. Stadtman, E.R., Protein oxidation and aging, *Science,* 257, 1220–1224, 1992.

50. Davies, K.J., Protein damage and degradation by oxygen radicals, *J. Biol. Chem.,* 262, 9895–9901, 1987.

51. Garner, M.H. and Spector, A., Selective oxidation of cysteine and methionine in normal and senile cataractous lenses, *Proc. Natl. Acad. Sci. USA,* 77, 1274–1277, 1980.

52. Marx, G. and Chevion, M., Site-specific modification of albumin by free radicals: reactions with copper (II) and ascorbate, *Biochem. J.,* 236, 397–400, 1986.

53. Yu, B.P., Cellular defenses against damage from reactive oxygen species, *Physiol. Rev.,* 74, 139–162, 1994.

54. Richter, C., Biophysical consequences of lipid peroxidation in membranes, *Chem. Phys. Lipids,* 44, 175–189, 1987.

55. Girotti, A.W., Mechanisms of lipid peroxidation, *Free Rad. Biol. Med.,* 1, 87–95, 1985.

56. Bielski, B.H., Arudi, R.L., and Sutherland, M.W., A study of the reactivity of hydrogen peroxide and superoxide anion with unsaturated fatty acids, *J. Biol. Chem.,* 258, 4759–4761, 1983.

57. Aust, S.D., Morehouse, L.A., and Thomas, C.E., Role of metals in oxygen radical reactions, *Free Rad. Biol. Med.,* 1, 3–25, 1985.

58. Corongiu, F.P., Poli, G., Dianzani, M.V., Cheesman, K.H., and Slater, T.F., Lipid peroxidation and molecular damage to polyunsaturated fatty acids in rat liver, *Chemico-Biol. Interact.,* 59, 147–155, 1986.

59. Reiter, R.J.R., Functional pleiotropy of the neurohormone melatonin: antioxidant protection and neuroendocrine regulation. *Frontiers Neuroendocrinol.,* 16, 383–415, 1995.

60. Poeggeler, B., Reiter, R.J.R., Tan, D.X., Chen, L.D., and Manchester, L.C., Melatonin, hydroxyl radical mediated oxidative damage, and aging: a hypothesis, *J. Pineal Res.,* 14, 141–168, 1993.

61. Reiter, R.J.R., Antioxidant properties of melatonin: a molecule conserved throughout the animal kingdom, *Verh. Dtsch. Zool. Ges.,* 87, 195–204, 1994.

62. Reiter, R.J.R., The pineal gland and melatonin in relation to aging: a summary of the theories and of the data, *Exp. Gerontol.,* 30, 199–212, 1995.

63. Reiter, R.J.R., Oxidative processes and antioxidative defense mechanisms in the aging brain, *FASEB J.,* 9, 526–533, 1995.

64. Tan, D.X., Chen, L.D., Poeggeler, B., Manchester, L.C., and Reiter, R.J.R., Melatonin: a potent, endogenous hydroxyl radical scavenger, *Endocrine J.,* 1, 57–60, 1993.

65. Chen, L.D., Tan, D.X., Reiter, R.J.R., Yaga, K., Poeggeler, B., Kumar, P., Manchester, L.C., and Chambers, J.P., *In vivo* and *in vitro* effects of the pineal gland and melatonin on [Ca^{2+},Mg^{2+}]-dependent ATPase in cardiac sarcolemma, *J. Pineal Res.,* 14, 178–183, 1993.

66. Pristos, C.A., Constantinides, D.P., Tritton, T.R., Heinbrook, D.L., and Sartorelli, A.C., Use of high performance liquid chromatography to detect hydroxyl and superoxide anion radicals generated by mytocyin C, *Ann. Biochem.,* 150, 294–299, 1985.

67. Towell, J. and Kalyanaraman, B., Detection of radical adducts of 5,5-dimethyl-1-pyroline-*N*-oxide by the combined use of high performance liquid chromatography with electrochemical detection and electron spin resonance, *Ann. Biochem.,* 196, 111–119, 1991.

68. Poeggeler, B., Saarela, S., Reiter, R.J.R., Tan, D.X., Chen, L.K., Manchester, L.C., and Barlow-Walden, L.R., Melatonin: a highly potent endogenous radical scavenger and electron donor. New aspects of the oxidation chemistry of this indole assessed *in vivo*, *Ann. N.Y. Acad. Sci.*, 738, 419–420, 1994.

69. Poeggeler, B., Reiter, R.J.R., Hardeland, R., Chen, L.D., Tan, D.X., Manchester, L.C., and Barlow-Walden, L.R., Radical scavenging ability of melatonin, in *Melatonin: Mechanismos de Accion e Implicaciones Tempeuticas*, abstr. 4, Curso Internacional, 1994.

70. Poeggeler, B., Reiter, R.J.R., Hardeland, R., Swernek, E., Melchiorri, D., and Barlow-Walden, L.R., Melatonin, a mediator of electron transfer and repair reactions, acts synergistically with the chain breaking antioxidants ascorbate, trolox, and glutathione, *Neuroendocrinol. Lett.*, 17, 87–92, 1995.

71. Hardeland, R., Reiter, R.J.R., Poeggeler, B., and Tan, D.X., The significance of the metabolism of the neurohormone melatonin: protection and formation of bioactive substances, *Neurosci. Biobehav. Rev.*, 17, 347–357, 1993.

72. Pieri, C., Marra, M., Moroni, F., Decchioni, R, and Marcheselli, F., Melatonin: a peroxyl radical scavenger more potent than vitamin E, *Life Sci.*, 55, 271–276, 1994.

73. Miller, J.A., Structure-activity studies of the carcinogenicities in the mouse and rat of some naturally occuring and synthetic alkenylbenzene derivatives related to safrole and estragole, *Cancer Res.*, 43, 1124–1134, 1983.

74. Randerath, K., Reddy, M.V., and Disher, R.M., Age and tissue related DNA modification in untreated rats: detection by ^{32}P-post-labeling assay and possible significance for spontaneous tumor induction and aging, *Carcinogenesis*, 7, 1615–1617, 1986.

75. Tan, D.X., Poeggeler, B., Reiter, R.J.R., Chen, L.D., Chen, S., Manchester, L.C., and Barlow-Walden, L.R., The pineal hormone melatonin inhibits DNA-adduct formation induced by the chemical carcinogen safrole *in vivo*, *Cancer Lett.*, 70, 65–71, 1993.

76. Littlefield, L.G., Joiner, E.E., Colyer, S.P., Sayer, A.M., and Frome, E.L., Modulation of radiation induced chromosome aberrations by DMSO, an OH radical scavenger. 1. Dose response studies in human lymphocytes exposed to 220 kV X-rays, *Int. J. Radiat. Biol.*, 53, 875–890, 1988.

77. Okada, S., Nakamura, N., and Sasaki, K., Radioprotection of intracellular genetic material, in Dygaard, O.F. and Simic, M.G., Eds., *Radioprotectors and Anticarcinogens*, Academic Press, New York, 1983, 339–356.

78. Vijayalaxmi., Reiter, R.J.R., Meltz, M.L., Melatonin protects human blood lymphocytes from radiation induced chromosome damage, *Mutat. Res.*, 346, 23–31, 1995.

79. Vijayalaxmi., Reiter, R.J.R., Sewerynek, E., Poeggeler, B., Leal, B.Z., and Meltz, M.L., Marked reduction in radiation induced micronuclei in human blood lymphocytes pretreated with melatonin, *Rad. Res.*, 143, 102–106, 1995.

80. Blinkinstaff, R.T., Brandstadter, S.M., Reddy, S., and Witt, R., Potential radioprotective agents. 1. Homologs of melatonin, *J. Pharmacol. Sci.*, 83, 216–218, 1994.

81. Abe, M., Reiter, R.J.R., Orhii, P.B., Hara, M., and Poeggeler, B., Inhibitory effect of melatonin on cataract formation in newborn rats: evidence for an antioxidative role for melatonin, *J. Pineal Res.*, 17, 94–100, 1994.

82. Spector, A. and Garner, W.H., Hydrogen peroxide and human cataract, *Exp. Eye Res.,* 33, 673–681, 1981.

83. Calvin, H.I., Medvendovsky, C., and Worgal, B.V., Near total glutathione depletion and age specific cataracts induced by buthionine sulfoximine in mice, *Science,* 223, 553–555, 1986.

84. Reiter, R.J.R., Craft, C.M., Johnson, J.E., Jr., King, T.S., Richardson, B.A., Vaughan, G.M., and Vaughan, M.K., Age associated reduction in nocturnal melatonin levels in female rats, *Endocrinology,* 109, 1295–1297, 1981.

85. Reiter, R.J.R., Richardson, B.A., Johnson, L.Y., Ferguson, B.N., and Dinh, D.T., Pineal melatonin rhythm: reduction in aging Syrian hamsters, *Science,* 210, 1372–1373, 1990.

86. Pierrefiche, G., Topall, G., Courbain, G., Henriet, I., and Laborit, H., Antioxidant activity in mice, *Res. Commun. Chem. Pathol. Pharmacol.,* 80, 211–223, 1993.

87. Melchiorri, D., Reiter, R.J.R., Attia, A.M., Hara, M., Burgos, A., and Nistico, G., Potent protective effect of melatonin on *in vivo* paraquat induced oxidative damage in rats, *Life Sci.,* 56, 83–89, 1994.

88. Ghezzi, P., Saccardo, B., and Bianchi, M., Role of reactive oxygen intermediates in the hepatotoxicity of endotoxin, *Immunopharmacology,* 12, 241–244, 1986.

89. Pentney, P. and Bubenik, G.A., Melatonin reduces the severity of dextran induced colitis in mice, *J. Pineal Res.,* 19, 31–39, 1995.

90. Wells, C.L. and Rhame, F.S., Effect of oral dextran sulfate on the mouse intestinal tract, *J. AIDS,* 3, 361–365, 1990.

91. Gross, V., Arndt, H., Andus, T., Palitzsch, K.O., and Scholnerick, J., Free radicals in inflammatory bowel diseases: pathophysiology and therapeutic implications, *Hepatogastroenterology,* 41, 320–327, 1994.

92. Valles, E.G., deCastro, C.R., and deCastro, J.A., *N*-acetyl cysteine is an early but not late preventive agent against carbon tetrachloride induced liver necrosis, *Toxicol. Lett.,* 71, 87–95, 1994.

93. Recknagel, R.O., Glende, E.A., Dolak, J.A., and Waller, R.L., Mechanisms of carbon tetrachloride toxicity, *Pharmacol. Ther.,* 43, 139–154, 1989.

94. Daniels, W.M., Reiter, R.J.R., Melchiorri, D., Sewerynek, E., Pablos, M.I., and Ortiz, G.G., Melatonin counteracts lipid peroxidation induced by carbon tetrachloride but does not restore glucose-6-phosphatase activity, *J. Pineal Res.,* 19, 1–6, 1995.

95. Sewerynek, E., Poeggeler, B., Melchiorri, D., and Reiter, R.J.R., Hydrogen peroxide induced lipid peroxidation in rat brain homogenates is greatly reduced by melatonin, *Neurosci. Lett.,* 195, 203–205, 1995.

96. Sewerynek, E., Melchiorri, D., Ortiz, G.G., Poeggeler, B., and Reiter, R.J.R., Melatonin reduces hydrogen peroxide induced lipid peroxidation in homogenates of different rat brain regions, *J. Pineal Res.,* 19, 51–56, 1995.

97. Chen, L.D., Melchiorri, D., Sewerynek, E., and Reiter, R.J.R., Retinal lipid peroxidation *in vitro* is inhibited by melatonin (unpublished).

98. Melchiorri, D., Reiter, R.J.R., Sewerynek, E., Chen, L.D., and Nistico, G., Melatonin reduces kainate induced lipid peroxidation in homogenates of different brain regions, *FASEB J.,* 9, 1205–1210, 1995.

99. Giusti, P., Lipartiti, M., Franceschini, D., Schiavo, N., Floreani, M., and Manev, H., Neuroprotection by melatonin from kainate induced excitotoxicity in rats, *FASEB J.,* 10, 891–896, 1996.

100. Mohan, N., Sadeghi, K., Reiter, R.J.R., and Meltz, M., The neurohormone melatonin inhibits cytokine, mitogen, and ionizing radiation induced NF-κB, *Biochem. Mol. Biol. Int.,* 37, 1063–1070, 1995.

101. Barlow-Walden, L.R., Reiter, R.J.R., Abe, M., Pablos, M., Menendez-Palaez, A., Chen, L.D., and Poeggeler, B., Melatonin stimulates brain glutathione peroxidase activity, *Neurochem. Int.,* 26, 497–502, 1995.

102. Gilad, E., Cuzzocrea, S., Zingarelli, B., Salzman, A., Szabo, C., Melatonin is a scavenger of peroxynitrite, *Life Sci.,* 60(10), PL169–PL174, 1997.

103. Pryor, W. and Squadrito, G., The chemistry of peroxynitrite: a product from the reaction of nitric oxide with superoxide, *Am. J. Physiol.,* 268, L699–L722, 1995.

104. Crow, J.P. and Beckman, J.S., The role of peroxynitrite in nitric oxide-mediated toxicity, *Curr. Topics Microbiol. Immunol.,* 196, 57–73, 1995.

105. Szabo, C., The pathophysiological role of peroxynitrite in shock, inflammation, and ischemia-reperfusion injury, *Shock,* 6, 79–88, 1996.

106. Sewerynek, E., Reiter, R.J.R., Melchiorri, D., Ortiz, G.G., and Lewinski, A., Oxidative damage in the liver induced by ischemic reperfusion: protection by melatonin, *Hepatogastroenterology,* 43, 898–905, 1996.

Chapter **4**

Antioxidant Activity of Melatonin as Assessed by Chemiluminescence

Alexander Ivanovich Kuzmenko

Contents

Mechanisms of the Non-Enzymatic Lipid Free-Radical Oxidation

Currently, much attention is being paid to investigation of the hormone melatonin as an antioxidant. The antioxidant influence of melatonin on the brain,[1] on cyanide-induced oxidation,[2] *in vivo*,[3] and *in vitro*[4] as well as its radioprotective effect[5] have been shown. Here we will deal with the mechanisms of its action as an antioxidant on non-enzymatic lipid or unsaturated fatty acid free radical oxidation.

Lipid oxidation begins with an initiation stage (see below). Initiators can be ionizing radiation action,[5] reactions leading to free radical formation (Fenton reaction[6]), or substances capable of decomposing with free radical generation.[7] After the initiation stage, the lipid free oxidation comes to the propagation stage and oxidation termination.[7,8]

Initiation: formation of R$^.$

Propagation: R$^.$ + O$_2$ $\longrightarrow$ ROO$^.$

ROO$^.$ + RH (substrate) $\longrightarrow$ ROOH + R$^.$

Decomposition: ROOH + Me^{2+} $\longrightarrow$ RO$^.$ + OH$^-$ + Me^{3+}

ROOH + Me^{3+} $\longrightarrow$ ROO$^.$ + H$^+$ + Me^{2+}

ROOH + ROOH $\longrightarrow$ ROO$^.$ + RO$^.$ + H$_2$O

Termination: R$^.$ + R$^.$ $\longrightarrow$ nonradical products

R$^.$ + ROO$^.$ $\longrightarrow$ nonradical products

ROO$^.$ + ROO$^.$ $\longrightarrow$ nonradical products

There are many low-molecular-weight substances with antioxidizing activity in free radical reactions. Thus, these low molecular substance are known as natural and synthetic antioxidants. One of the most investigated natural antioxidants is vitamin E. According to the theory of free radical oxidation, its antioxidizing activity is stipulated by its participation in reaction with free radicals.[9] The rate constants of the α-tocopherol reaction with linoleic acid is $(24.2 \pm 4.2) \times 10^4$ M^{-1} sec^{-1} in homogeneous solution and $(1.59 \pm 0.20) \times 10^4$ M^{-1} sec^{-1} in the membrane at 30°C.[10]

The presence of mobile hydrogen in the α-tocopherol-hydroxy group leads to the vitamin E antioxidizing property. The rate constant for hydrogen abstraction from α-tocopherol by poly(peroxysteryl)peroxil radicals in water is about 3.2×10^6 M^{-1} sec^{-1} at 30°C.[11] The α-tocopherol reactions with peroxil radicals are observed in the following reactions:[9]

AoOH + ROO$^.$ $\longrightarrow$ AoO$^.$ + ROOH

AoO$^.$ + ROO$^.$ $\longrightarrow$ nonradical combination products

This type of antioxidant is known as a phenolic antioxidant. There are many synthetic antioxidants synthesized by analogs to vitamin E.[11] For example, Trolox (synthetic analog of the vitamin E) is widely used as an antioxidant. The other class of the antioxidants is the amines, which have a mobile hydrogen in the amino group, also, and can react with a lipid peroxyl radical.[12]

So, the availability of mobile hydrogen in the hydroxy or amino group in the structure of antioxidants is highly desirable. In regard to the molecular structure of melatonin, it does not contain a hydroxy or amino group, as do some other indole derivatives such as serotonin. The absence of the hydroxy group in the melatonin carbon atom in the 5 position and the absence of the amino group in the carbon side chain found in serotonin probably lead to melatonin's lesser antioxidizant property or antioxidant activity at higher concentrations. Actually, the antioxidizing activity of serotonin is exhibited at a concentration of 0.03 mM.[13] An equal effect for melatonin was observed at a tenfold higher concentration.[13]

Much experimental data about the antioxidizing action of melatonin exists;[13–15] however, the melatonin molecule has no classic antioxidizing center, and its mechanisms differ from the antioxidizing actions of other classic antioxidants. One of the reactional centers in the melatonin molecule which may be responsible for its antioxidizing property is the nitrogen atom in the indole ring and its hydrogen. In his research, Reiter[15,16] showed the cation radical formation at this nitrogen atom and the mechanisms of its cation formation.[16]

Possible Mechanisms of the Melatonin Antioxidizing Action

The melatonin antioxidizing mechanism differs from classic antioxidant action. To understand the antioxidant effect of melatonin, it would be helpful to investigate other mechanisms, such as:

1. Synergy of other antioxidant actions
2. Substances capable of changing the membrane structure
3. Complex formations with other antioxidants and their transportation up to and into the membrane
4. Chelators of the biometal

Now we are going to consider in detail these methods of further research.

Low-molecular-weight substances are well known to have the ability to strengthen the action of other antioxidants.[17] The mechanism of this phenomenon is an antioxidant radical reduction up to the initial condition.[18] In organisms and in their biological membranes, the natural antioxidants are always present. The melatonin antioxidizing effect *in vivo* and *in vitro* can consist in strengthening already existing antioxidant actions. The antioxidizing effect of melatonin synergistically increases in the presence of ascorbate, Trolox, or glutathione.[19] The action can be verified *in vitro* in an artificial model. It is possible to create a homogeneous[11] or heterogeneous[20] system from clean, unsaturated fatty acids or lipids: without an antioxidant, with an antioxidant, with melatonin, or with a combination of melatonin and an antioxidant in identical concentrations. It is likely that the actions of melatonin and of some of its antioxidant compositions will be more effective than their effects without melatonin.

The other important factor affecting lipid oxidation in membrane is their fluidity. Changes in the fluidity of membranes enable natural antioxidant penetration into membranes, as well as free radicals generated from outside of a membrane. Free radical oxidation of membranes has been found to decrease with a decrease in their fluidity.[21] A substance capable of stabilizing the membrane will influence the ability of lipids or fatty acids to oxidize in these membranes indirectly. As recently shown, melatonin is capable of changing the fluidity of membranes.[13] Based upon the data of Daniels et al.,[13] introduction of 1.0×10^5 M melatonin statistically reduced the microviscosity of membranes. The supposition is offered that melatonin is located in the membrane between bilayers. The other substance with an indole structure — serotonin — is located inside a bilayer and has no such effect on membrane fluidity.[13] To determine how melatonin interacts with a membrane is possible, as it has been shown for sterols.[22]

It is important to keep in mind that the influence of biometals (Fe, Cu, etc.) on lipid free radical oxidation is essential.[23] It is well known that iron can react with hydrogen peroxide by the Fenton reaction.[6] The OH· radical formed in the Fenton reaction is capable of reacting with lipid and polyunsaturated fatty acids at the initiation stage.[24] Iron can also participate in alkyl peroxide[23] or lipid peroxide decomposition.[8] High iron levels in an animal's diet have been shown to decrease vitamin E and to increase lipid free radical oxidation,[25] thus the iron plays an essential role at some critical stage.[26] Iron and copper deficiencies also lead to other disorders.[27,28]

Melatonin has the ability to react with hydroxyl and peroxyl radicals. The rate constants of these reactions are 6.0×10^{10} M^{-1} sec^{-1} and 7.5×10^{10} M^{-1} sec^{-1}, respectively.[29] It is possible to determine the influence of melatonin on lipid peroxide decomposition and the formation of peroxyl radicals in the presence of ion transitive metal, as well as in the chemical and biochemical model of lipid or unsaturated fatty acid oxidation.

Recently, the search for new metal chelators as substances capable of terminating the lipid free radical oxidation has intensified.[30,31] Deferoxamine can chelate iron,[32] and thioctic acid is capable of copper chelation.[31] There are many other chelators available for medicinal applications.[33] The indole can form similar complexes with such metals as Na^+, K^+, and Li^+.[34] The complexes between indole structures and transition metals are known.[35] It is suggested that melatonin, as an indol structure substance, is capable of such complex formation with iron or copper in an organism. It can be proven in lipid-metal containing systems, as has been shown for liposomes.[30,31]

Herbich et al.[36] have shown that substances with indol structures (including melatonin) are capable of hydrogen bond formation. In this case, the hydrogen bond formation between the indole and the phenolic antioxidant hydroxy group is possible. Because melatonin is a water- and lipid-soluble substance,[13] the opportunity for antioxidant transport up and into the biological membrane arises. The same kind of transportation is known for α-tocopherol.[37] On the other hand, the possibility of a hydrogen bond with the antioxidant hydroxy group will prevent its spontaneous spending.

Application of Chemiluminescence for Melatonin Antioxidant Activity Testing

In the majority of cases, melatonin antioxidizing activity is measured by malondialdehyde determination.[1–4,38] The malondialdehyde level is measured by the thiobarbituric acid test. Malondialdehyde is a final product of lipid oxidation.[7,26] It is impossible to estimate by malondialdehyde determination the influence of melatonin as an antioxidant in the early stages of lipid oxidation. This method is based on thiobarbituric acid reactions with aldehydes formed as a result of lipid free radical oxidation. Many authors note that this is not only malondialdehyde definition, but that all thiobarbituric acid-reactive substances are being determined.[39] Moreover, this fact complicates discussion of experimental results. At the present time, it is known that other aldehydes (not only malondialdehyde) play an essential role in lipid oxidation. Malondialdehyde can influence membrane microviscocity.[40]

In a lipid free radical oxidation investigation, in order to avoid the drawbacks described above, the chemiluminescence method application can be used. This method provides the opportunity to measure free radicals directly during their formation. Vladimirov et al.[41] have shown, that chemiluminescence is observed in the lipid peroxyl radical reaction. The chemiluminescence method offers the chance to determine free radicals directly to investigate melatonin antiradical activity. Unlike chemiluminescence, determining thiobarbituric acid-reactive substances assesses only the antioxidizing properties of melatonin.

The sensitivity of the chemiluminescence method is quite high. For example, chemiluminometer PChL-01 (State Scientific Research Institute of Biological Engineering, Russia) has a sensitivity of 1×10^5 quantum/sec $\times 4\pi$. It enables determination of lipid free radical oxidation in microbiological tests. This is very important for practical use in applied medicine, especially in pediatrics research. Lipid free radical oxidation determination by the chemiluminescence test is carried out at a temperature of 37°C.[41] In contrast, the thiobarbituric acid-reactive product determination requires heating to a temperature higher than physiological.[39] The chemiluminescence determination is carried out in physiological solution (NaCl or some buffers system).[42] This is very important for lipid oxidation determination in cells, tissues homogenates, or biological fractions. Unlike lipid peroxide determination, preliminary extraction by cyclohexane and diethyl esther is required.[43] Some other methods require an ethanol solution.[44] These organic solvents are capable of influencing lipid free radical oxidation.[45]

One other benefit of the chemiluminescence method is important to mention. It is an unremitting lipid free radical oxidation determination from the moment of its initiation to the end of the biological testing; therefore, the chemiluminometer 1254-001 Luminova (Bio-Orbit Oy, Finland) permits registration of the chemiluminescence signal each second. The chemiluminometer PChL-01 (State Scientific Research Institute of Biological Engineering, Russia) has the ability to register chemiluminescence signals even more frequently.

The chemiluminescence method enables determination of various stages of the lipid free radical oxidation. For example, lipid peroxide decomposition, after the introduction of iron, is observed in the first minute and general lipid oxidation 3 to 5 minutes later.[42] Also, some kinetic parameters correlate with malondialdehyde quantity or thiobarbituric acid-reactive substances in oxidizing samples.[41] Some parameters allow evaluation of the lipid oxidation rate, and the activity of antioxidants has been measured in research.[41] The variety of the experimentaly determined chemiluminescence kinetical parameters provides the opportunity to reveal the influence of melatonin at various stages of lipid free radical oxidation. It is possible that the antioxidant reduces the quantity of lipid peroxides, the first lipid free radical oxidation stable product, yet has no influence on accumulation of aldehydes, a final product of lipid oxidation.

It is significant to note that chemiluminescence determination requires a small period of time for measurement. Depending upon the methodology applied, a period of from 3 to 4[42,46] or up to 10 minutes[41] is sufficient. This difference in time necessary for the tests is closely connected with the kind of sample (tissue or blood). Certainly, analysis time depends on the initiator which is applied (H_2O_2, Fe^{2+}, azocompounds). The quantity of natural antioxidants in the test sample is important, too. More antioxidant content in the sample requires more time for determination of lipid free radical oxidation. As an example, for one thiobarbituric acid-reactive substances determination, 60 minutes are necessary.[39] Futhermore, the chemiluminescence method uses a small quantity of biological material for the analysis. If the chemiluminescence determination is made in tissue homogenate or biological fractions, 1 to 2.5 mg/ml of the protein are required.[42] For one test determination,[47] 75 to 100 µl of blood are enough. This is an important feature for dynamic lipid free radical oxidation monitoring of experimental animals or for patients such as small children, as only a small quanitity of blood needs to be drawn from the finger.

Finally, but not last, there is the possibility for process automation. Any chemiluminometer can be connected to a computer. The chemiluminescence curve is equal to chromatographic (signal measurement at the time). This fact offers a chance to use electronic equipment which already exists. By applying computer equipment, it is possibe to register quickly various stages of the chemiluminescence process which would otherwise be impossible in a hand-operated mode. Computer equipment allows the automatic calculation of many kinetical chemiluminescence parameters, which will minimize the impact of individual researchers on designated parameters. Application of computer techniques allows storage of experimental data and subsequent analysis of that data.

In conclusion, it may be said that the antioxidant and antiradical influence of melatonin on lipid free radical oxidation is not yet clear. Research has indicated that melatonin is an antioxidant;[1-5,13-16] however, its complex antioxidant properties require systematic investigation in diverse directions. For determining the antioxidizing and antiradical properties of melatonin, the chemiluminescence method is applicable. With the chemiluminescence method, it is possible to determine the influence of melatonin on the various stages of lipid free radical oxidation *in vivo* and *in vitro*. The high sensitivity of the chemiluminescence method gives the opportunity to reveal the minimum quantity of melatonin necessary for an antioxidizing effect.

Acknowledgment

We thank Anna Je. Plistchenko for technical assistance in preparation of this manuscript.

References

1. Melchiorri, D., Reiter, R.J., Sewerynek, E., Chen, L., and Nistico G., Melatonin reduces kainate-induced lipid peroxidation in homogenates of different brain regions, *FASEB J.*, 9, 1205, 1995.

2. Yamamoto, H. and Tang, H., Preventive effect of melatonin against cyanide-induced seizures and lipid peroxidation in mice, *Neurosci. Lett.*, 207, 89, 1996.

3. Melchiorri, D., Reiter, R.J.R., Attia, A.M., Hara, M., Burgos, A., and Nistico, G., Potent protective effect of melatonin on *in vivo* paraquat-induced oxidative damage in rats, *Life Sci.*, 56, 83, 1995.

4. Sewerynek, E., Melchiorri, D., Chen, L., and Reiter, R.J.R., Melatonin reduces both basal and bacterial lipopolysaccharide-induced lipid peroxidation *in vitro, Free Radic. Biol. Med.*, 19, 903, 1995.

5. Vijayalaxmi, Reiter, R.J.R., Sewerynek, E., Poeggeler, B., Leal, B.Z., and Meltz, M.L., Marked reduction of radiation-induced micronuclei in human blood lymphocytes pretreated with melatonin, *Radiat. Res.*, 143, 102, 1995.

6. Fenton, H.J.H., Oxidation of tartaric acid in the presence of iron, *J. Chem. Soc.*, 65, 899, 1994.

7. Bartosz G., *Druga Tward Tlenu*, Wudawnictwo Naukowe PWN, Warszawa, 1995, 95.

8. Rice-Evans, C.A. and Diplock A.T., Techniques in free radical research, in Burdon R.H. and van Knippenberg P.H., Eds., *Laboratory Techniques in Biochemistry and Molecular Biology,* Vol. 22, Elsevier, New York, 1991, 40.

9. Huang, S., Frankel, E.N., and German, J.B., Antioxidant activity of α- and γ-tocopherols in bulk oils and in oil-in-water emulsions, *J. Agric. Food Chem.*, 42, 2108, 1994.

10. Barclay, L.R.C., Baskin, K.A., Locke, S.J., and Schaefer, T.D., Benzophenone-photosensitized autoxidation of linoleate in solution and sodium dodecyl sulfate micelles, *Can. J. Chem.*, 65, 2529, 1987.

11. Valgimigli, L., Ingold, K.U., and Lusztyk, J., Antioxidant activities of vitamin E analogues in water and a Kamlet-Taft b-value for water, *J. Am. Chem. Soc.*, 118, 3545, 1996.

12. Melvin, J.Yu., McCowan, J.R., and Phebus, L.A., Benzylamine antioxidants: relationship between structure, peroxyl radical scavenging, lipid peroxidation inhibition and cytoprotection, *J. Med. Chem.*, 36, 1262, 1993.

13. Daniels, W.M.U., Rensburg S.J., Zul, J.M., Walt, B.J., and Taljaard, J.J.F., Free radical scavenging effects of melatonin and serotonin: possible mechanism, *NeuroReport*, 7, 1593, 1996.

14. Reiter, R.J.R., Pablos, M.I., Agapito T.T., and Guerrero J.M., Melatonin in the context of the free radical theory of aging, *Ann. N.Y. Acad. Sci.*, 786, 362, 1996.

15. Reiter, R.J.R., Antioxidant action of melatonin, *Adv. Pharmacol.*, 38, 103, 1997.

16. Reiter, R.J.R., Functional diversity of the pineal hormone melatonin: its role as an antioxidant, *Exp. Clin. Endocrinol.*, 104, 10, 1996.

17.   Girotti, A., Mechanisms of lipid peroxidation, *J. Free Radic. Biol. Med.,* 1, 87, 1985.

18.   Barclay, L.R.C., Dakin, K.A., and Zahalka, H., Ascorbate: antioxidant activity determination in a hydrocarbon phase using quaternary ammonium salts as phase-transfer agents, *Can. J. Chem.,* 70, 2148, 1992.

19.   Poeggeler, B., Reiter, R.J.R., Hardeland, R., Sewerynek, E., Melchiorri, D., and Barlow-Walden, L.R., Melatonin, a mediator of electron transfer and repair reaction, acts synergistically with the chain-breaking antioxidant ascorbate, Trolox and glutathione, *Neuroendocrinol. Lett.,* 17, 87, 1995.

20.   Barclay, L.R.C. and Vinquvist, M.R., Membrane peroxidation: inhibiting effects of water-soluble antioxidants on phospholipids of different charge types, *Free Radic. Biol. Med.,* 16, 779, 1994.

21.   Shimada, K., Okada, H., Matsuo, K., and Yoshioka, S., Involvement of chelating action and viscosity in the antioxidative effect of xanthan in an oil/water emulsion, *Biosci. Biotech. Biochem.,* 60, 125, 1996.

22.   Duval, D., Durant, S., and Homo-Delarche, F., Interaction of steroid molecules with membrane structure and function, *Biochim. Biophys. Acta.,* 737, 409, 1983.

23.   Aust, S.D., Morehouse, L.A., and Thomas, C.E., Role of metals in oxygen radical reactions, *Free Radic. Biol. Med.,* 1, 3, 1985.

24.   Aruoma, O.I., Characterization of drugs as antioxidant prophylactics, *Free Radic. Biol. Med.,* 20, 675, 1996.

25.   Dabbagh, A.J., Mannion, T., Lynch, S.M., and Frel, B., The effect of iron overload on rat plasma and liver oxidant status *in vivo, Bichem. J.,* 300, 799, 1994.

26.   Aruoma, O.I., Free radicals and antioxidant strategies in sports, *J. Nutr. Biochem.,* 5, 370, 1994.

27.   Olsson, K.S., Marsell, R., Ritter, B., Olander, B., Akerblom, A., Ostergard, H., and Larsson, O., Iron deficiency and iron overload in Swedish male adolescents, *J. Internal Med.,* 237, 187, 1995.

28.   Chen, Y., Saari, J.T., Kang, Y.J., Weak antioxidant defenses make the heart a target for damage in copper-deficient rats, *Free Radic. Biol. Med.,* 17, 529, 1994.

29.   Poeggeler, B., Reiter, R.J.R., Hardeland, R., Tan, D.X., and Barlow-Walden, L.R., Melatonin and structurally related, endogenous indoles act as potent electron donors and radical scavengers *in vitro, Redox Rep.,* 2, 179, 1996.

30.   Rachidi, S., Coudray, C., Baret, P., Gelon, G., Pierre, J., and Favier, A., Inhibition of lipid peroxidation by a new family of iron chelators, *Biol. Trace. Elem. Res.,* 41, 77, 1994.

31.   Ou, P., Tritschler, H.J., and Wolff, S.P., Thioctic (lipoic) acid: a therapeutic metal-chelating antioxidant?, *Biochem. Pharmacol,* 50, 123, 1995.

32.   Shatrov, V.A., Boelaert, J.R., Chouaib, S., Droge, W., and Lehmann,V., Iron chelation decreases human immunodeficiency virus-1 Tat potentiated tumor necrosis factor-induced NF-κB activation in Jurkat cells, *Eur. Cytokine Netw.,* 8, 37, 1997.

33.   Hider, R.C., Porter, J.B., and Singh, S., The design of therapeutically useful iron chelators, in *The Development of Iron Chelators for Clinical Use,* Bergeron, R.J. and Brittenham, G.M., Eds., CRC Press, Boca Raton, FL, 1994, 353.

34. Brown, R.T., Jouli, J.A., and Sammes, P.G., Indoles, in Sammes, P.G., Ed., *Comprehensive Organic Chemistry,* Vol. 8, Pergamon Press, New York, 1979, 752.

35. Melendez, E., Merchan, F.L., Tejero, T., Merino, P., and Garcia, M., Synthesis of 2,2'-(alkylenediamino)dibenzazoles: new heterocyclic tetradentate ligands, *Ann. Quim.,* 90, 487, 1994.

36. Herbich, J., Hung, C., Thummel, R.P., and Waluk J., Solvent-controlled excited state behavior: 2-(2'-pyridyl)indoles in alcohols, *J. Am. Chem. Soc.,* 118, 3508–3518, 1996.

37. Mowri, H., Nakagawa, Y., Jnoue, K., and Nojima, E., Enhancement of the transfer of α-tocopherol between liposomes and mitochondria by rat-liver protein(s), *Eur. J. Biochem.,* 117, 537, 1981.

38. Giusti, P., Franceschini, D., Petrone, M., Manev, H., and Floreani, M., *In vitro* and *in vivo* protection against kainate-induced excitotoxicity by melatonin, *J. Pineal Res.,* 20, 226, 1996.

39. Ohkawa, H., Ohishi, N., and Yagi, K., Assay for lipid peroxides in animal tissues by thiobarbituric acid reaction, *Anal. Biochem,* 95, 351, 1979.

40. Buko, V., Artsukevich, A., Maltsev, A., and Shareyko, S., Modification of rat liver membranes by aldehydic end-products of lipid peroxidation, *Curr. Top. Biophys.,* 18, 195, 1994.

41. Vladimirov, Yu.A. and Archakov, A.I., *Lipids Peroxidation in Biological Membranes,* Nauka, Moscow, 1972, 252 (in Russian).

42. Kuzmenko, A.I., Morozova, R.P., Nikolenko, I.A., Korniets, G.V., and Kholodova, Yu.D., Effect of vitamin D_3 and ecdysterone on free radical lipid peroxidation, *Biochemistry (Moscow),* 62, 609, 1997.

43. Zhang, D., Yasuda, T., Yu, Y., Zheng, P., Kawabata, T., Ma, Y., and Okada, S., Gunseng extract scavenges hydroxyl radical and protects unsaturated fatty acids from decomposition caused by iron-mediated lipid peroxidation, *Free Radic. Biol. Med.,* 20, 145, 1996.

44. Tsuda, T., Mizuno, K., Ohshima, K., Kawakishi, S., and Osawa, T., Supercritical carbon dioxide extraction of antioxidative components from Tamarind (*Tamarindus indica* L.) seed coat, *J. Agric. Food Chem.,* 43, 2803, 1995.

45. Vladimirov, Yu.A., Sherstnev, M.P., and Azimbaev, T.K., Estimation of antioxidative and antiradical activity of substances and biological objects by means of iron-initiated chemiluminescence, *Biophysics,* 37, 1041, 1992.

46. Kimura, H. and Nakano, M., Highly sensitive and reliable chemiluminescence method for the assay of superoxide dismutase in human erythrocytes, *FEBS Lett.,* 239, 347, 1988.

47. Goode, H.F., Richardson, N., Myers, D.S., Howdle, P.D., Walker, B.E., and Webster, N.R., The effect of anticoagulant choice on apparent total antioxidant capacity using three different methods, *Ann. Clin. Biochem.,* 32, 413, 1995.

Chapter 5

Muscle, Metabolism, and Melatonin

John C. George

Contents

Introduction

Movement is the most visible manifestation of life and its cessation of death. Be it of the lowly amoebae or of the multitudes of diverse animals in water, on land, or in the air, their modes of locomotion form an essential part of their capacity for survival. Muscle, besides providing the power for locomotion and performance of work, is also a major source of metabolic heat which not only enhances muscular efficiency but also provides body heat for a homeotherm to survive in a cold environment. Muscle has the capacity for generating heat quickly by shivering when the body is

0-8493-8564-4/99/$0.00+$.50

exposed to cold. Ectothermic vertebrates, such as lizards, bask in sunshine to raise body temperature so as to enhance the efficiency of muscles in foraging activity. Many insects, such as butterflies, grasshoppers, and dragonflies, also bask in sunshine for preflight warm-up. Nocturnal moths, dragonflies, and bees are capable of contracting their flight muscles to produce metabolic heat by shivering like endothermic vertebrates.[1] The ability of bees to produce heat quickly by shivering so as to elevate their own body temperatures and thereby that of their nests, as well, was a physiological acquisition that significantly contributed to their survival.

Traditionally, human activities such as athletics and the use of animals such as horses, reindeers, dogs and pigeons in racing competitions created considerable interest in exercise physiology with a view to improving muscular performance. In recent years, however, there has been a surge of research activity in exercise physiology and nutritional studies due to increasing public awareness of the need for maintaining high levels of physical fitness and well-being, largely based on the mounting evidence that regular exercise reduces the prevalence of coronary disease.

The pigeon as a laboratory animal model has, over the years, contributed substantially to our present knowledge of muscle physiology and energy metabolism. Indeed, the very foundations of modern knowledge of aerobic metabolism were laid by the early observations of Szent-Gyorgyi that minced pigeon breast muscle could oxidize pyruvate completely, provided catalytic amounts of dicarboxylic acids such as succinate, fumarate, malate, and oxaloacetate were added. These findings ultimately led to the important discovery of the tricarboxylic acid cycle (Krebs cycle) by Hans Krebs, using the same tissue preparation.[2] Building on these foundations, the present discourse will deal with aspects of the role of the pineal gland and of its hormone, melatonin, in the regulation of muscular activity and metabolic homeostasis.

Muscle Fiber Types and Metabolic Adaptation

The discovery of the Krebs cycle and its significance in metabolic pathways stimulated studies on the cellular organization and metabolic adaptation of the component fiber types of the pigeon breast muscle. It was shown that the pigeon breast muscle (M. pectoralis pars thoracis) consists of two distinct fiber types: (1) a less numerous, broad, white type lacking myoglobin and intracellular lipid droplets and containing relatively smaller and fewer mitochondria, but rich in glycogen and glycolytic enzymes, thus adapted for anaerobic metabolism utilizing carbohydrate as fuel; and (2) a substantially more numerous, narrow, red, myoglobin- and lipid-loaded type containing numerous large mitochondria rich in oxidative enzymes, thus adapted for aerobic metabolism, metabolizing lipid as the main fuel (Figure 1).[3-6] It was shown that the red muscle fibers could metabolize fatty acids as fuel for muscular energy and that in migratory birds fat is the major source of energy for their long and sustained flights.[5,7-9] However, initially, glycogen is utilized by the white fibers, as in take-off and during the initial part of flight. As flight continues, there is a shift to fat utilization by the red fibers, which are well equipped for aerobic metabolism.

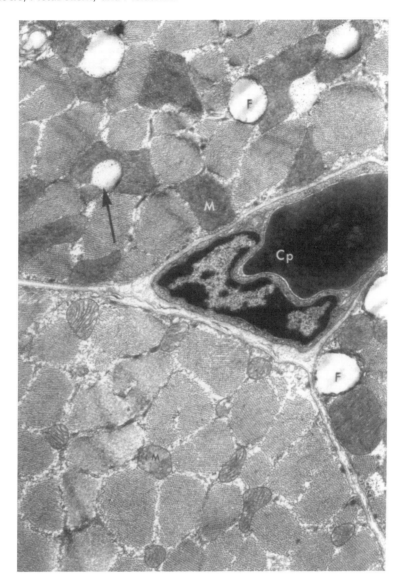

FIGURE 1
Electron micrograph of the pigeon breast muscle. Transverse section showing (top) red fiber, (middle right) blood capillary (cp) and part of another red fiber, and (bottom left) white fiber. Fat droplets (F) are seen only in the red fiber, one of which is partly engulfed by a mitochondrion (arrow). (Original magnification ×17,000.) (From Grinyer, I. and George, J.C., *Can. J. Zool.*, 47, 517, 1969. With permission.)

During cruising flight, the glycogen content of the white fibers is replenished to be used in short-term activity when needed, as in quick changing of flight direction.[5,9,10] When the bird is exposed to cold, the white fibers have been found to have a major role in shivering thermogenesis.[11]

Interest was thus generated in regard to the cellular organization and characterization of the fiber types of mammalian skeletal muscles.[12–17] In both avian and mammalian skeletal muscles, the occurrence of an intermediate fiber type was recognized.[5,14,17] Greater precision in fiber typing became possible with the development of new histochemical, immunohistochemical, and histophysiological techniques. Studies were directed toward obtaining a more comprehensive and unifying characterization of muscle fiber types combined with their metabolic profiles.[18–20] In adult mammalian muscles, a slow-twitch (type I) and two fast-twitch (type IIA and type IIB) types were identified. Intermediate forms of type II were recognized as type IID.[21] By combining the metabolic profile and functional performance, types I, IIA, and IIB are considered synonymous with types SO (slow-oxidative), FOG (fast-oxidative-glycolytic), and FG (fast-glycolytic), respectively.[18,21] In those mammals that are relatively less active, muscles contain high proportions of type IIB fibers, while those bred for races either for speed or endurance show different profiles in fiber composition.[22,23]

The red (FOG) and white (FG) fibers of the pigeon breast muscle correspond to the mammalian muscle types IIA and IIB, respectively. The FOG fibers are adapted for sustained fast contractions, metabolizing primarily fat as fuel to generate energy (adenosine triphosphate, ATP). The pectoralis of all birds capable of flapping flight consist predominantly of this type, whereas FG fibers, when present, are adapted for short-term, explosive, flapping flight, metabolizing glycogen as fuel to generate ATP. In some species, an intermediate FOG subtype, as in the pectoralis of starlings, replaces the original FG type but functions as FG fibers.[24] In birds such as sparrows and hummingbirds, the pectoralis consists of only one fiber type, FOG, corresponding to the red fibers. Slow fibers are present in very few numbers within a small narrow strip of muscle called the deep red strip found in the pectoralis of a few species such as chicken, Japanese quail, etc.[24,25] In the pectoralis of flightless birds such as the emu and ostrich, there exists a substantially higher proportion of slow fibers.[26]

It has been shown in mammalian muscles that the contractile and metabolic characteristics could be altered by changing their nervous innervation. The motor nerve from the slow soleus muscle of the cat was surgically made to innervate the fast flexor digitorum longus and the nerve of the latter muscle to innervate the former. This cross innervation resulted in the slow muscle becoming a fast muscle and vice versa in contrast to the contralateral control muscles.[27] Concomitant with changes in contractile characteristics of the cross-innervated muscles, there were also changes in the metabolic profile of their fiber types. The slow muscle showed a decrease in oxidative activity with simultaneous increase in glycolytic enzyme activity, whereas the fast muscle acquired greater oxidative enzyme activity and lower glycolytic enzyme activity.[28,29] Experiments have also shown that changes in muscle could be brought about by inducing changes in the nature of activity without changing innervation.[29] Activity that requires speed (such as sprint running) tended to increase fiber diameter and also glycolytic metabolism.[29,30] It is known that race horses and greyhounds, even before they commence training for races, have different muscle fiber composition,[31] thereby indicating that some individuals may already have been endowed with the physical basis for a particular type of activity so that with definitive training they could be expected to excel with greater certainty than for the others. For example, some may have a predominance of type I muscle fibers and could be good candidates to be trained as long-distance runners, while those with a predominance of type IIB fibers could be trained as sprinters. These are possibilities worthy of consideration for future research.

The Pineal and Locomotor Activity

The daily cycle of alternating light and darkness associated with the Earth's rotation acts as a powerful environmental cue for the establishment of an endogenous circadian rhythm which functions as the body's time-keeping mechanism or "biological clock". Diurnal animals remain active in the daytime and sleep during the night, whereas nocturnal ones do the opposite. During the period of activity, their body temperature remains higher than during the period of inactivity. The pineal acts as the intermediary between the external environment and the endocrine system of the organism. In mammals, the nervous signals generated by the cyclic environmental lighting are transmitted to the pineal via its sympathetic nerves. As a response to darkness or the absence of light input, the pineal synthesizes its hormone, melatonin (N-acetyl-5-methoxytryptamine, MT), which has been termed "the chemical expression of darkness" by Reiter.[32] This "Dracula" hormone, MT, is then released into the bloodstream. By virtue of the pineal's capacity to respond to the nervous signals generated by cyclic environmental lighting and to convert that information to a hormonal signal, the pineal has been called a photoneuroendocrine transducer.

In the synthesis of MT, the primary precursor, tryptophan, an essential amino acid which cannot be synthesized by the body, is converted to serotonin, which in turn is converted to N-acetylserotonin by the rate-limiting enzyme, N-acetyltransferase.[33] N-acetylserotonin is then methylated to MT by the enzyme hydroxyindole-O-methyltransferase (HIOMT).[34,35]

In a study to explore the influence of the pineal on locomotor activity rhythm, Gaston and Menaker[36] observed in house sparrows that the removal of their pineal glands abolished their normal circadian rhythm of perch-hopping locomotor activity. When the pineal glands were implanted from donor sparrows into the anterior chamber of the eye of the pinealectomized (Pxd) sparrows, the circadian perch-hopping rhythm was re-established with the time-setting of the donor sparrows.[37] It was also shown that, in addition to the locomotor activity, the body temperature (T_b) rhythm was also abolished by pinealectomy (Pxy).[38] Single MT injections (1.2 to 2.5 mg) produced a reduction in T_b of 4.7°C in sparrows.[39–41]

That Pxy abolished free-running locomotor rhythms has been shown in other passerine birds, too;[42–45] however, Pxy failed to abolish circadian rhythm in the Japanese quail[46] and the pigeon.[47] It was observed that when pigeons maintained under a 12L:12D photocycle were Pxd and bilaterally enucleated, the circadian rhythm of circulating levels of MT was completely abolished, but not when they were only Pxd. Of the nighttime peak of blood-borne MT, 70% was found to have come from the pineal, whereas only 17 and 13% were contributed by the retina and other sources, respectively.[48] As was demonstrated by Oshima et al.,[49] when pigeons were Pxd as well as blinded, the rhythms of both locomotor activity and T_b were abolished.

Abolition of circadian activity rhythms by Pxy did not occur in some other vertebrate classes of animals (e.g., reptiles[50] and mammals[51]). It is known that all members of the reptilian subclass Archosauria lack pineal bodies. However, non-pineal MT is present in the blood of *Alligator mississippiensis*.[52] Though the absence of a distinct pineal gland has been reported in the nine-banded armadillo, *Dasypus novemcinctus*, a clear diurnal rhythm of circulating levels of MT has been found in this animal.[53] The above observations do indicate that the pineal gland is not the only source of MT in the body and that the discrepancies with regard to the failure of Pxy to abolish circadian rhythms in certain species reported in the literature could be attributed to the presence of extrapineal MT in the body. Indeed, MT has been shown to be present at several other sites in the body (see Chapter 2, this volume).

In man, there is considerable evidence to show that MT production in the pineal is influenced by the daily light/dark cycle and that MT may have a significant role as mediator of certain cyclic events.[54-56] In studies investigating the effect of exogenous MT administration in humans, the problem of the existing endogenous MT rhythm is seldom considered. This aspect has been projected by Petterborg et al.[57] in their study of a patient lacking endogenous MT caused by ablation of his pineal in the course of radiation treatment for pineal astrocytoma.

The Pineal and Temperature Regulation

Light and temperature are two important environmental factors that influence organisms and their circadian and seasonal activities. The seasonal activities of animals that are influenced by these environmental cues are mainly reproduction, migration, and hibernation. Substantial evidence has accumulated that strongly suggests that MT produced by the pineal gland has a regulating role in the reproductive activity of seasonally breeding mammals[58] (see Chapter 12, this volume). Melatonin has also been implicated in the production of body changes such as seasonal obesity in animals (see Chapter 7, this volume). However, little is known regarding the role of the pineal or its hormone, MT, in the premigratory fattening in migratory birds or the winter fattening in birds inhabiting the temperate zone. It has been observed in broiler chicks that Pxy caused loss in body weight and impaired efficiency of energy retention, whereas administration of exogenous MT increased body weight and energy retention.[59] On the other hand, in a study on Japanese quail fed MT in drinking water, Zeman et al.[60] reported a decrease in abdominal fat deposition, in total lipids in the breast muscle, and triacylglycerols in plasma, indicating an inhibitory effect of MT on lipogenesis. In an ultrastructural study of the seasonal changes in the pineal gland of the migratory Canada goose, the authors[61] indicated the existence of a structural basis for the cyclic seasonal activity of the gland. Assessing the overall activity of the pineal on the basis of cellular and nuclear size, the abundance of mitochondria, ribosomes, microtubules, and dense-core vesicles, the spring postmigratory phase had the highest pineal activity. During this period (early May), the ambient temperature (T_a) at the breeding grounds at Fort Churchill in the subarctic region of Manitoba (Canada) was the lowest ($-12°$ to $-3°C$) among all the periods studied. Based on the amount of ribosomes, size, and/or number of mitochondria and the presence of Golgi complex and/or microtubules, the breeding, spring, and fall premigratory phases showed high pineal activity. However, when judging the secretory activity of the pineal by the presence of secretory granules in transendothelial transport, the spring and fall premigratory phases appeared to be the most active.[61] That the premigratory phase in the annual life cycle of a migratory bird is the period of fattening in preparation for migration has been well documented.[5] This process of fattening is influenced by environmental factors such as light, temperature, and humidity and is controlled by processes of metabolic and hormonal regulation.[62] In the process of building up energy reserves, catabolic processes have to be toned down and anabolic processes enhanced. This is illustrated in a study involving the capacity for fatty acid oxidation of the breast muscle of a migratory starling during its premigratory period and that of a non-migratory starling during the same period.[7] Possibly the role of MT is to tone down metabolism. The influence of MT in the promotion of growth in birds has been suggested by previous authors.[59,63–65] It has also been reported[66] that MT increases serum levels of growth hormone and insulin-like growth factor I in male Syrian hamsters. In light of the above observations, MT rhythm in the life of an organism functions both as a clock and a calendar, as proposed by Reiter.[67]

During the molting period (late July/early August), the Canada goose sheds all of its flight feathers and becomes flightless. At this time of the year, T_a is about $10°C$ at the breeding grounds.[61] The bird has to cope with this low temperature with much reduced body insulation. It has been shown in the pigeon that when it is exposed to cold ($-25°C$) with some feathers plucked from the breast area, the bird experiences severe cold stress and goes into a shivering frenzy.[11] On the other hand, when a bird is exposed to heat, the problem it faces is to dissipate the excess body heat so as to maintain normal T_b. It has been shown in winter pigeons that Pxy causes hyperthermia and, when MT is implanted subcutaneously, T_b is brought down to normal (Figure 2).[68,69] Though Pxy caused hyperthermia, the circadian T_b rhythm was not affected when the pigeons were kept in either $25°$ or $3°C$ T_a for 2 or 3 weeks. However, when pigeons were exposed to $-18°C$ T_a for 280 min, there was a marked drop in T_b in all the three groups of pigeons — namely, Pxd, sham-operated, and normal. Yet, the Pxd pigeons did register a T_b higher than that of the other two groups during the photophase but not in the scotophase. The failure of the hyperthermic effect of Pxy to show up during the scotophase in pigeons exposed to acute cold ($-18°C$) T_a for 280 min indicated that the thermoregulatory role of the pineal was not effective at $-18°C$ during the scotophase. This effect was attributed to low thyroid activity in the scotophase, as it is known in man that circulating levels of thyroxine (T_4) and triiodothyronine (T_3) are low during the night.[70] The reversal of the hyperthermic effect of Pxy by MT has been explained as being due to MT inducing vasodilation for dissipation of heat.[69]

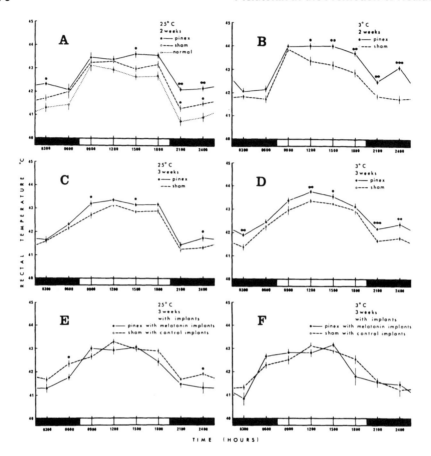

FIGURE 2

Circadian rhythm in cloacal temperature (mean °C ± SE) (T_b) in the pigeon. (A) and (B) show the effect of pinealectomy on T_b following a 2-week postsurgical acclimation to 25 and 3°C, respectively, and (C) and (D) show the same following a 3-week acclimation to 25 and 3°C, respectively. (E) and (F) show the effect of melatonin implantation on pinealectomized pigeons, acclimated to 25 and 3°C for 3 weeks. The dark area on the horizontal axis represents scotophase and clear area the photophase. * $p < 0.05$; ** $p < 0.01$; *** $p < 0.001$ (when compared to respective controls). Pinex = pinealectomized. (From John, T.M., Itoh, S., and George, J.C., *Hormone Res.*, 9, 41, 1978. With permission.)

Subsequently, however, when T_b in the Pxd and control pigeons was monitored after 2 weeks, it was found that there was no difference in T_b between the two groups. The pigeons showed no difference in T_b even the next winter.[71] By repeating the experiments with summer pigeons, it was observed that Pxy did not produce the significant hyperthermia obtained with winter Pxd pigeons. The obliteration of hyperthermia after a lapse of postsurgery period in Pxd winter pigeons and in Pxd summer pigeons was attributed to a possible supply of MT from extra-pineal sources. It was also observed that there was an apparent decrease in foot temperature (T_f) in Pxd winter and fall pigeons, thereby suggesting that the hyperthermia in these pigeons was due to reduced heat dissipation.[71] The foot in birds is known to be a major site for heat dissipation.[72–74] These observations indicate the importance of environmental factors such as photoperiod and temperature in experimental studies seeking to investigate the role of MT in the body.[75–80] It is therefore important to recognize that parameters such as T_f in birds and (in the case of mammals) tail temperature in rats[81] and ear temperature in rabbits also have to be monitored. In this regard, reports of thermoregulatory responses to MT administration in different mammalian species have been varying. For example, Arutyunyan et al.[82] observed in mice a depression of 2° to 3°C in T_b following injection of MT, whereas Barchas et al.[83] obtained no effect in rabbits. However, MT counteracted the hyperthermic effect of amphetamine. The action of MT on T_b may also depend on the site of injection. A slight increase in T_b was produced in rats when MT (60 mg) was injected into the cerebral ventricles of the brain, whereas intraperitoneal injections caused significant rise in T_b,[84] which suggests a central action for MT depending on the feedback from peripheral tissues.

Melatonin has been implicated in inducing torpor in the white-footed mouse.[85] Administration of MT has also been found to induce, as well as cause prolonged hibernation in, the ground squirrel.[86] Prolonged exposure to cold has been shown to induce in mammals hypertrophy of the brown adipose tissue (BAT),[87] which is the major effector of non-shivering thermogenesis in the cold-adapted rat.[88] Heldmaier and Hoffman[89] observed that subcutaneous implantation of MT in Djungarian hamsters induces hypertrophy of BAT. These observations indicate the influence of photoperiod and temperature and its effect on the pineal and BAT. This is in accord with the findings of Reiter[90] in the female golden hamster in that the hypertrophy of BAT, stimulated by exposing the animal to long scotophase, is prevented by Pxy. However, Pxy was found to have no effect on diet-induced thermogenesis and BAT proliferation in rats.[91]

The pineal gland has also been shown to have a significant role in the thermoregulatory behavior of ectothermic lower vertebrates. In fish, Pxy causes disruption of diel rhythms of behavioral thermoregulation and leads them to select a markedly elevated T_a.[92] The diel rhythm of the oxygen consumption of frogs was abolished after the pineal eye was removed.[93] The removal of the photoreceptive parietal eye caused lizards to seek higher T_a.[94]

Due to the growing interest in the importance of the pineal gland and its hormone, MT, in thermoregulation in vertebrates,[68,69,78,92–97] including man,[98] efforts were directed toward locating MT receptors in the target tissues of the body. Detection of pharmacologically specific binding sites for MT became possible when Vakkuri et al.[99] first synthesized 2-[^{125}I] iodomelatonin (I-MT). Using I-MT, Vanecek et al.[100] identified hypothalamic MT binding sites in the rat. It has been postulated that in mammals the carotid *rete* served as a brain-cooling system in which blood travels to the circle of Willis after losing some of the heat to the pool of cooler venous blood.[101] As mentioned earlier, blood flow to the tail in the rat serves as a means of heat dissipation.[81,102] The same may be expected to occur in the peripheral circulation of animals that do not have a prominent tail. Heat dissipation in those animals could take place via extremities and certain parts of the body such as the human forearm and finger, hind limb of the baboon, flippers in marine mammals, feet in birds, or ears in rabbits.

Using I-MT, Viswanathan et al.[103] localized, characterized, and validated the function of specific MT receptors in the smooth muscle layer of the caudal artery and the anterior cerebral artery forming the circle of Willis in the rat. That these arterial binding sites are functional MT receptors in the caudal artery of the rat was demonstrated by producing norepinephrine-induced contractions of the caudal artery *in vitro* potentiated by MT.[103] Evans et al.[104] were able to show that MT could act directly when vasoconstrictor activity of isolated segments of the caudal artery from juvenile rats was tested under 60 mmHg pressure. The greater expression of vascular MT receptors observed in young rats is indicative of the greater need for thermoregulation in young ones in which a higher body surface area/volume ratio exists. This vasoconstriction response was not seen in adult rats, which is in agreement with the observation of Laitinen et al.[105] that the MT receptor expression in the caudal artery of rats declines with age (for reviews on MT binding sites,[106,107] see Chapter 1, this volume).

The vasoconstrictor expression of MT-receptors in the rat caudal artery strips was revealed only after pretreatment with norepinephrine.[103] This suggests that, when circulating levels of endogenous MT are high, there would be vasoconstriction of the caudal artery causing reduction in blood flow and less heat loss. Such a response to MT would be important to the animal in the night when T_a is lower and MT levels in the blood are high. However, in rats subjected to voluntary overfeeding with a highly palatable diet (cafeteria diet), causing increased thermogenesis, T_b was maintained by increased heat dissipation from the tail as indicated by increased tail skin temperature (T_t). No effect on T_t or BAT deposition was seen in Pxd rats, thereby suggesting that the pineal has no direct involvement in modulating the metabolism of BAT in the rat.[91] In birds, unlike in mammals, BAT is absent and catecholamines, especially norepinephrine which has high calorigenic action in mammals exposed to cold, have been observed to produce dose-dependent hypothermia in cold exposed pigeons.[80,108,109] When MT-implanted (MI) pigeons were exposed to cold (Figure 4), it was found that T_f was significantly greater than that in the controls, indicating increased heat dissipation from the feet.[108] In this context it should be mentioned that Weekley[110] reported that MT caused dose-dependent relaxation of precontracted (30 mM KCl) vascular smooth muscle in the rat aorta, indicating that MT per se has the capacity to relax vascular smooth muscle. However, this observation relates to relatively large vessels such as the thoracic aorta and may not be applicable to changes occurring in the capillaries. Obviously, we need to know more about the actual mechanism of MT action in thermoregulation.

Melatonin and Metabolism

Antiquity and Obiquity of Melatonin

The history of MT probably has its beginnings from the time of the origin of organismic life itself. Melatonin is the most dynamic endogenous mediator of photoperiodic information in organisms from algae to humans or, perhaps, its structurally related tryptophan metabolites in all organisms.[111,112] As a highly diffusible lipophilic molecule, MT could penetrate all cellular membranes and act as a fine tuner of physiological events.[113] The antiquity of MT and other tryptophan-derived indoles may be traced to the origin of photosynthetic organisms producing massive amounts of oxygen which enabled others to utilize the readily available natural oxidant for respiration and metabolism.[114] The occurrence of pineal indoleamines at very low levels of phylogeny in the evolutionary scale has been recorded.[115,116] With the increase in aerobic metabolism in organisms, there also came the need for a molecule with antioxidant capacity to protect cells from the damaging effects of oxidative stress. It has been suggested that the initial function of MT was to detoxify the free radicals formed from molecular oxygen[117] (see also Chapter 3, this volume).

As for the ubiquity of MT, besides being present in all the various organisms studied,[112] in the vertebrates MT has been located in several tissues besides the pineal[118] (see also Chapter 2, this volume).

Metabolic Responses to Melatonin

In the previous section, MT was shown to have a hypothermic role in the thermoregulation of pigeons. In this section we will discuss the metabolic responses to MT, as indicated by cloacal (body) temperature (T_b), foot temperature (T_f), shivering activity, heart rate (HR), breathing frequency (BF), and oxygen consumption (VO_2), monitored in MT-implanted (MI) pigeons exposed to T_a gradually dropping from 34°C to 2°C.[108] The MI pigeons maintained throughout a lower T_b than the control (MC) pigeons (Figure 3). This is consistent with the earlier observation that MT implantation nullifies or reverses the hyperthermic effect of Pxy,[68,69] and also with the observation that T_f in Pxd pigeons was lower than in the control, indicating lower heat dissipation due to less circulating levels of MT.[119] The role of MT was thus indicative of being a facilitator of vasodilation and increased blood flow so as to enhance peripheral heat dissipation. It can be seen in Figure 4 that both MC and MI pigeons showed gradual decreases in T_f in response to drop in T_a. The decrease in T_f in MI pigeons appeared to be less pronounced than that in the MC pigeons, as T_a dropped below 20°C, but the drop in T_b was not statistically significant.[108]

The intensity of shivering activity in both groups of pigeons increased after T_a fell to 26°C, but the rate of shivering was relatively slow in MI pigeons (Figure 5).[108] The lower shivering intensity in MI pigeons was attributed to the hypothermic action of MT. It was also suggested that the action of MT was due to effecting a lower setpoint centrally and increasing vasodilation peripherally. Studies on mammals have indicated that MT receptors are present in the brain, particularly in the region of the medial preoptic and the suprachiasmatic areas.[120] The peripheral vasodilatory action of MT has been shown in its capacity for lowering the vasoconstrictor effects induced by various constrictor agents in Pxd rats.[121]

Consistent with the envisaged role of MT in toning down metabolism, both HR and BF in MI pigeons were lower than in MC pigeons (Figures 6 and 7).[108] With

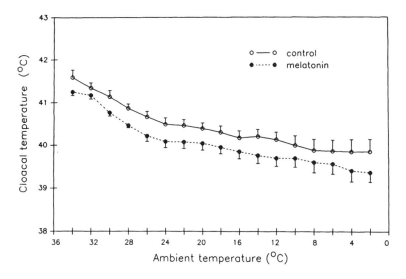

FIGURE 3

Cloacal temperature (T_b) in control (MC) and melatonin-implanted (MI) pigeons exposed to ambient temperature (T_a) gradually reduced from 34°C to 2°C. MC vs. MI: $p = 0.000$; T_a effect: $p = 0.000$; interaction: $p = 1.000$; n = 8 MC and 8 MI. (From John, T.M. and George, J.C., in Riklis, E., Ed., *Photobiology,* Plenum Press, New York, pp. 597–605, 1991. With permission.)

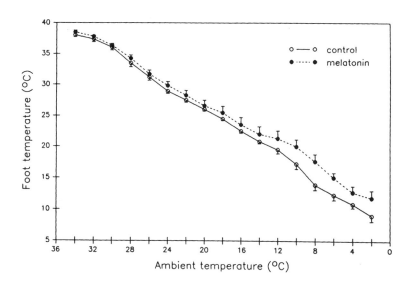

FIGURE 4

Foot temperature (T_f) in MC and MI pigeons exposed to T_a, as in Figure 3. MC vs. MI: $p = 0.000$; T_a effect: $p = 0.000$; interaction: $p = 0.525$; n = 8 MC and 8 MI. (From John, T.M. and George, J.C., in Riklis, E., Ed., *Photobiology,* Plenum Press, New York, pp. 597–605, 1991. With permission.)

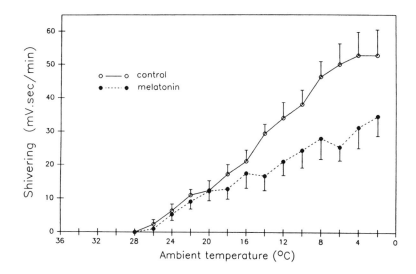

FIGURE 5

Shivering in MC and MI pigeons exposed to T_a, as in Figure 3. MC vs. MI: $p = 0.000$; T_a effect: $p = 0.000$; interaction: $p = 0.0289$; n = 7 MC and 7 MI. (From John, T.M. and George, J.C., in Riklis, E., Ed., *Photobiology*, Plenum Press, New York, pp. 597–605, 1991. With permission.)

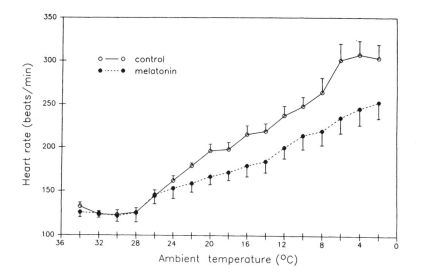

FIGURE 6

Heart rate (HR) in MC and MI pigeons exposed to T_a, as in Figure 3. MC vs. MI: $p = 0.000$; T_a effect: $p = 0.000$; interaction: $p = 0.033$; n = 8 MC and 8 MI. (From John, T.M. and George, J.C., in Riklis, E., Ed., *Photobiology*, Plenum Press, New York, pp. 597–605, 1991. With permission.)

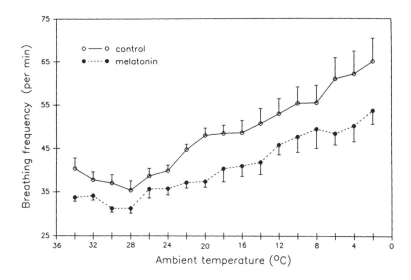

FIGURE 7

Breathing frequency (BR) in MC and MI pigeons exposed to T_a, as in Figure 3. MC vs. MI: $p = 0.000$; T_a effect: $p = 0.000$; interaction: $p = 0.910$; n = 8 MC and 8 MI. (From John, T.M. and George, J.C., in Riklis, E., Ed., *Photobiology*, Plenum Press, New York, pp. 597–605, 1991. With permission.)

lower T_a below 28°C, HR in both groups of pigeons increased, as expected, but that of the MI pigeons remained lower than that of the MC ones. As for BF, the increase was registered in both groups below T_a of 28°C but, again, BF was lower throughout in the MI pigeons.[108] As for VO_2, there was an increase in both groups below T_a of 28°C (Figure 8).[108] However, VO_2 in the MI pigeons showed a trend to be slightly lower than that in MC pigeons, particularly below a T_a of 12°C, though the difference was not statistically significant. With the significantly lower BF, HR, and shivering activity in MI pigeons, one would have expected to see significantly lower VO_2 as well. Perhaps in the avian body, which lacks BAT and for which shivering is the only way for quick thermogenesis when exposed to cold, it becomes imperative that VO_2 should not be drastically reduced in order to survive. This is probably achieved by maintaining a steady blood T_3/T_4 ratio. It has been observed in MI pigeons that, while circulating levels of T_4 were significantly reduced, the T_3/T_4 ratio was maintained at a significantly higher level than that in MC pigeons.[65] It is possible that there is active peripheral monodeiodination occurring in MI pigeons.

Melatonin and Muscular Activity

Fuel of Muscle Metabolism

The three fiber types (I, IIA, and IIB), each metabolically adapted for functioning at different levels of performance, were discussed above. In most human locomotor

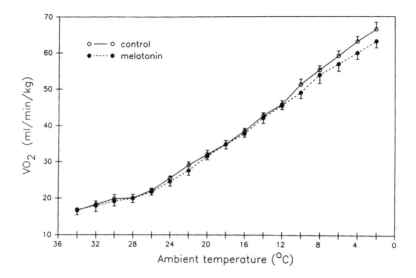

FIGURE 8

Oxygen uptake (VO_2) in MC and MI pigeons exposed to T_a, as in Figure 3. MC vs. MI: $p = 0.016$; T_a effect: $p = 0.000$; interaction: $p = 0.994$; n = 7 MC and 7 MI. (From John, T.M. and George, J.C., in Riklis, E., Ed., *Photobiology*, Plenum Press, New York, pp. 597–605, 1991. With permission.)

muscles, all the three types are present. Depending on the action of the muscle, one type may be more numerous than the other two. Red muscles, which primarily use fat as fuel to generate ATP for energy, consists predominantly of type I fibers. In the muscles of long-distance runners, type I fibers are more numerous than the others. Marathon runners are known to have 80% type I fibers in most of their leg muscles.[122] It is reported that Alberto Salazar, who won the 1982 Boston marathon, had over 90% type I fibers in his leg muscles.[122] On the other hand, sprinters metabolizing glycogen have a high type II fiber content (76%) in their leg muscles.[122]

The main storage of glycogen in the body is in the skeletal muscles and the liver, whereas fat is stored mainly in the adipose tissue, even though fat in the form of intracellular droplets occurs in type I fibers (Figure 1). It has been estimated that if a single fuel were to be used, 100% of liver glycogen and 100% of muscle glycogen would be exhausted in 20 and 70 min, respectively, during muscular exercise, whereas 50% of the adipose tissue triglyceride fatty acids would last for 400 min during a marathon race.[122] This indicates that no one fuel is adequate to meet the energy demands of marathon racing.[122] One gram of triglyceride would yield 35 kJ of energy, while the same amount of glycogen would yield only 16 kJ.[122] Also, triglycerides as fuel would yield considerably more metabolic water than carbohydrate; however, in the utilization of fat, oxygen is an absolute necessity, whereas glycogen and glucose could be metabolized anaerobically by glycolysis. It should be mentioned here that skeletal muscle forms the main reservoir of protein during starvation. During starvation, it is the myofibrillar proteins that are primarily affected. As a result of the protein breakdown, the amino acids released could be

TABLE 1
Effects of Anesthesia (Sodium Pentobarbital) and Exercise on Daytime Circulating Levels of Melatonin (pg/ml serum) in the Pigeon

Normal (Resting)	Under Anesthesia (Resting) (1 hr)	Under Anesthesia (Breast Muscles Exercised by In Vivo Electrical Stimulation) (1 hr)	After 48 km Free Flight (60–80 min)
26.48 ± 5.38 (9)[a]	66.57 ± 23.08 (7)[b]	75.39 ± 20.77 (7)[c]	48.22 ± 7.64 (11)[d]

Note: Figures in parentheses denote number of birds used. Values are mean ± SEM. Differences between a, b: significant; b, c: not significant; a, d: significant; $p < 0.05$. There was no significant change in plasma/serum osmolality.

Source: Data compiled from John et al.[124,125]

converted to glucose in the liver by the process known as gluconeogenesis. Muscle protein breakdown could also occur during and after a long-distance race.[122]

Melatonin and Metabolic Regulation

Single intravenous injections of exogenous MT given to resting pigeons have shown that plasma levels of glucose[63] and free fatty acids[123] (when given in the scotophase) and growth hormone[63] (when MT was given in the photophase) were increased. Chronic implantation of MT in pigeons produced an increase in plasma levels of glucose and growth hormone during daytime when MT levels are known to be lower than during night. However, the antithyroid action of MT was indicated by the decrease in the levels of T_4.[65] Serum levels of growth hormone have also been found to increase in male Syrian hamsters after MT administration.[66]

The above observations led to studies on changes in circulating levels of MT in exercised pigeons. The breast muscles of pigeons under anesthesia (sodium pentobarbital) were electronically stimulated via the brachial plexus of nerves for 1 hr.[124] Serum MT levels in the anesthetized birds were significantly higher than those in the normal birds, whereas MT levels in the anesthetized and those of the exercised ones were not significantly different (Table 1).[124,125] The markedly higher MT levels in the anesthetized birds compared to the normal values could be attributed to the action of the anesthetic drug in inducing sleep. However, it could be argued that MT acts as mediator of the drug, sodium pentobarbital, and the induced sleep is actually caused by the higher circulating levels of MT. Indeed, MT has been suggested as a mediator of atypical antipsychotic drug effects.[126]

It has been observed that, in pigeons and budgerigars during sustained flight, the heat produced in the body amounted to more than eight times the heat generated at rest.[127] In a study with homing pigeons, it was observed that after a natural free flight of 48 km lasting 60 to 80 min, there was about an 82% increase in the circulating levels of MT.[125] By virtue of the known hypothermic action on MT,[68,69,108] this daytime flight-induced increase in blood levels of MT should be considered as a mechanism to facilitate peripheral heat dissipation and thereby reduce the flight-induced heat-load.

In humans, a daytime increase in circulating levels of MT, β-endorphin, and cortisol resulting from a 28.5-mile mountain race has been reported.[128] It has been estimated that the rate of heat production during a marathon could be more than 1 kW, or at least 13 times greater than at rest.[122] A marathon runner, therefore, has to cope with the problem of increasing heat-load, which could lead to hyperthermia and heat stroke. It has been reported that, in the Empire Games in Canada in 1954, the British marathon runner Jim Peters collapsed in the final 400 m due to heat stroke; a British cyclist, Tony Simpson, died of heat stroke in the Tour de France in 1959; and Alberto Salazar was near death due to heat stroke after the Falmouth (MA) road race in 1978.[122] Therefore, a marathoner's need for sufficient rest and sleep in order to generate an adequate supply of MT cannot be overemphasized. Proper diet which enhances MT synthesis also requires serious consideration. It has been shown that a meal rich in carbohydrate could enable the brain to produce more serotonin, a precursor of MT, by increasing the uptake of tryptophan, an essential amino acid which in turn is a precursor of serotonin.[129] It is also important to know whether the pineal is the only source of the MT that is mobilized in the body to prevent the extreme threat of hyperthermia. Because the pineal is known not to store large amounts of MT,[130] one has to look for other sources of supply. It is possible that the large demands for MT would have to be met from extra-pineal sources. The gastrointestinal tract as a source of MT appears to be the best candidate to meet this demand (see Chapter 2, this volume).

Studies with laboratory mammals have shown that MT also has an analgesic action (see Reference 125 for a review). Exercise has been found to increase plasma levels of β-endorphin in humans.[131,132] In the migratory Canada goose, a marked reduction in β-endorphin-like immunoreactivity (β-ELI) observed in the pituitary during the spring and fall postmigratory periods has been attributed to being flight-induced.[133] This observation, that there was increased β-ELI in the pituitary prior to migration, correlates well with the finding of a corresponding increase in pineal secretory activity.[61]

It was mentioned earlier that during or after a long-distance race, there could be damage to muscle cells, thus causing muscle protein breakdown. Muscle fiber necrosis occurring in human marathon runners has been reported.[134] In the Canada goose after spring migration, degenerative changes such as Z-line streaming, mitochondrial loss, and presence of lipofuscin bodies have been described.[135] Similar exercise-induced changes in human muscle have been reported as well (for review, see Reference 135). Atrophy of muscle due to immobilization caused by injury is common in athletes. During molt, when the Canada goose loses its flight feathers and becomes flightless, the pectoral muscles undergo atrophy due to disuse while the leg muscles go into hypertrophy caused by overuse. The atrophic changes in the breast muscles are, however, followed by reparative and regenerative changes.[135]

Among vertebrates, birds represent the ultimate in aerobic life. The Cuban bee hummingbird (*Mellisuga helenae*) is the smallest homeotherm nature has produced. It is 5 cm in length and weighs 2.5 g. Much of the energy in a hummingbird is utilized to maintain its metabolic rate during the day, and during night it tends to go into torpor. During its annual migration, the ruby-throated hummingbird (*Archilochus colubris*) flies across the Gulf of Mexico, a distance of 500 miles, on a supply of 2 g of fat at a flight speed estimated to be 25 miles per hour.[5] Its breast muscles represent the highest level of adaptation for aerobic metabolism.[136] It would be of considerable interest to know the circulating levels of MT in a hummingbird before and after flight. High levels of MT would also be the answer for preventing oxidative damage due to high aerobic metabolism, as proposed by Reiter and associates.[117,137] There is also evidence to suggest the importance of other antioxidants such as uric acid in aerobic muscular activity. Circulating levels of uric acid were found to be significantly increased in homing pigeons after flight.[138,139] It was postulated that the flight-induced increase in blood levels of uric acid could also have a role in preventing flight-induced hyperthermia.[138,139]

While an increase in circulating levels of MT resulting from prolonged aerobic muscular activity has been clearly demonstrated in several studies,[125,128] there is no evidence for any such change in short-term intense activity. In fact, it has been shown that blood MT levels in men after completion of a 100-yard dash did not change, which suggests that the metabolic demands were insufficient to bring about a change in MT levels.[140]

Increased adrenocortical secretion is generally regarded as a stress response. In a study with homing pigeons, Haase et al.[141] observed that flights of less than 1 min duration and also of 315 to 561 min duration produced an increase in plasma levels of corticosterone. In another study with homing pigeons, Viswanathan et al.[142] observed that during a flight of 60 to 80 min there was no change in corticosterone levels. This leads to the conclusion that initially there is a rise in corticosterone levels which then levels off to rise again when flight is extended too long (for review, see Reference 139). It is possible that the reduction in circulating levels of corticosterone after the initial rise at the beginning of the flight might have been reduced by the increasing levels of MT.[125,139] There is evidence from a study with the Japanese quail that exogenous MT reduces plasma levels of corticosterone.[60]

Women, Exercise, and Amenorrhea

Blood levels of MT have been measured in women during the course of the menstrual cycle. In the morning, MT was low (34 pg/ml) on the 12th (preovulatory phase) and 25th day of the cycle, and was high (45 to 52 pg/ml) on the 22nd (luteal phase) and 4th day of the cycle.[41] In young women, during prolonged vigorous exercise, circulating levels of MT have been found to increase markedly.[143,144] It has also been observed that women athletes tend to be vulnerable to irregular menstrual cycles which may end up in total cessation of menstruation, a condition called amenorrhea. When it occurs in women runners, it is often referred to as "athletic amenorrhea". It has been suggested that there is a correlation between body fat level and the onset of amenorrhea.[122] Adequate body fat deposition is essential for child-bearing functions. In athletic amenorrhea, fat utilization has been increased to such an extent that the fat level goes down below the critical level. Hence, athletic amenorrhea has been found to be more common in the leanest women athletes who have acquired much endurance, in comparison to others. According to Newsholme and Leech,[122] in order to avoid this condition, the woman athlete should increase her body fat by increasing her energy intake by increasing carbohydrate intake of bread, potatoes, cereals, etc. rather than fat, which could create other undesirable problems. Such a diet would also ensure increased uptake of tryptophan, the building block of MT.[129]

In women patients with hypothalamic amenorrhea, an approximately threefold increase in nocturnal MT secretion has been reported.[145] From studies with animals, MT has been shown to inhibit hypothalamic gonadotropin-releasing hormone (GnRH)[146] and GnRH-induced elevation of intracellular Ca^{2+}.[147] Endogenous opioids present in excess in athletes[132,148] may enhance MT secretion and thereby produce more effective inhibition of GnRH. It has been observed that the inhibition by MT of GnRH-induced release of luteinizing hormone (LH) acts by inhibiting the production of cAMP.[149] In a study on the thermal and metabolic responses to cold in men and eumenorrheic and amenorrheic women, it was observed that amenorrheic women are more insensitive to cold than men or eumenorrheic women.[150] This is in accord with the finding that amenorrheic women have high blood levels of MT due to prolonged vigorous exercise[143,144] and also with the suggestion made earlier that the action of MT was due to effecting a lower set-point centrally and by increased vasodilation peripherally.

The pathophysiology of gonadal dysfunction in amenorrhea needs to be better understood. Adrenal hypertrophy and decreased levels of gonadal hormones as a result of strenuous exercise have been demonstrated in rodents; in amenorrheic women, higher plasma levels of cortisol, β-LPH and β-endorphin and also decreased levels of gonadotropin levels have been reported (for review, see Reference 151). From the above observations, it seems clear that amenorrhea is a stress response. Perhaps it is also the body's way of preventing unsafe pregnancy.

This multipotent molecule, MT, present in all organisms, plant and animal, has the elusive quality of a legend of long ago. In the vertebrates, it acts as a mulifunctional hormone, as a regulator of locomotor activity and sleep, of reproduction, migration, and hibernation. It regulates body temperature, metabolism, and immune functions. Perhaps it is a regulator of regulators. It has antisenescent and onchostatic properties. It also protects the body from oxidative stress and acts as a free radical scavenger. Is MT the conceptual *Amrit* (ambrosia, elixir) of Hindu mythology?

Summary

Skeletal muscles which form the physical basis of locomotor activity consist of fibers which are characterized by their metabolic adaptation and contractile properties.

Fibers which indulge in long-term activity are adapted for aerobic metabolism, metabolizing mainly fat as fuel, and those involved in fast short-term activity are adapted for anaerobic metabolism utilizing glycogen and glucose as fuel. A marathon runner has considerably more of the aerobic fibers in his leg muscles, whereas a sprinter's leg muscles consist predominantly of the anaerobic fibers. Similarly, in the case of a migratory bird, its powerful breast muscles are either predominantly or all aerobic fibers. Animals have a daily cycle consisting of a period of activity and one of inactivity (sleep) which is modulated by the pineal gland. This gland acts as a photoneuroendocrine transducer regulating the endogenous daily rhythm. Its hormone (MT) is synthesized and released into the blood stream. In diurnal animals, the circulating levels of MT are high during the night and low in the daytime. It is a sleep-inducing hormone and functions as a metabolic regulator, as well. During intense long-term muscular activity, circulating levels of MT have been found to increase significantly. In marathon runners after the race, as well as in homing pigeons after flight, increases in blood levels of MT have been documented. During long-term exercise, considerable amounts of heat are generated in the body, and MT acts as an endogenous antipyretic in order to offset the hyperthermia and thereby prevent a heat stroke. No such increase in MT levels has been noticed in short-term exercise such as a 100-yard sprint, as there is no thermal challenge involved. Women athletes often experience amenorrhea, presumably due to the high blood levels of MT which inhibit the release of the gonadotropin-releasing hormone, causing menstruation to cease during the period of athletic activity. Amenorrhea may be regarded as the body's physiological response to stress, ensuring the prevention of unsafe pregnancy. Melatonin has also been reported to possess antioxidant, antisenescent, and onchostatic properties.

Acknowledgments

I am deeply indebted to Dr. Paul D. Hebert, Chairman, Department of Zoology, University of Guelph, for providing facilities for work, and to Irene Teeter for typing the manuscript.

References

1. Heinrich, B., *Bumblebee Economics*, Harvard University Press, Cambridge, MA, 1979, 57.

2. Krebs, H.A., *Chemical Pathways of Metabolism*, Academic Press, New York, 1954.

3. George, J.C. and Naik, R.M., Relative distribution and chemical nature of the fuel store of the two types of fibres in the pectoralis major muscle of the pigeon, *Nature*, 181, 709, 1958.

4. George, J.C. and Talesara, C.L., A quantitative study of the distribution pattern of certain oxidizing enzymes and a lipase in the red and white fibres of the pigeon breast muscle, *J. Cell. Comp. Physiol.*, 58, 253, 1961.

5.   George, J.C. and Berger, A.J., *Avian Myology*, Academic Press, New York, 1966.

6.   Grinyer, I. and George, J.C., An electron microscopic study of the pigeon breast muscle, *Can. J. Zool.*, 47, 517, 1969.

7.   George, J.C. and Iype, P.T., Fatty acid oxidation by breast muscle homogenates of a migratory and non-migratory starling, *Pavo*, 2, 84, 1964.

8.   George, J.C. and Vallyathan, N.V., Capacity for fatty acid oxidation by the breast muscle of the starling (*Sturnus roseus*) in the pre- and post-migratory periods, *Can. J. Physiol. Pharmacol.*, 42, 447, 1964.

9.   Parker, G.H. and George, J.C., Effect of exercise on the respiratory metabolism of [1-^{14}C] palmitate-labeled pigeons, *Int. J. Biochem.*, 5, 167, 1974.

10. Parker, G.H. and George, J.C., Effects of short- and long-term exercise on intracellular glycogen and fat in pigeon pectoralis, *Jpn. J. Physiol.*, 25, 175, 1975.

11. Parker, G.H. and George, J.C., Glycogen utilization by the white fibres in the pigeon pectoralis as the main energy process during shivering thermogenesis, *Comp. Biochem. Physiol.*, 50A, 433, 1975.

12. George, J.C. and Susheela, A.K., A histo-physiological study of the rat diaphragm, *Biol. Bull.*, 121, 471, 1961.

13. Padykula, H.A. and Gauthier, G.F., Cytochemical studies of adenosinetriphosphatases in skeletal muscle fibers, *J. Cell Biol.*, 11, 87, 1963.

14. Ogata, T. and Mori, H., Histochemical study of oxidative enzymes in vertebrate muscle, *J. Histochem. Cytochem.*, 12, 171, 1964.

15. Gauthier, G.F. and Padykula, H.A., Cytological studies of fiber types in skeletal muscle. A comparative study of mammalian diaphragm, *J. Cell Biol.*, 28, 333, 1966.

16. George, J.C., Evolution of the bird and bat pectoral muscles, *Pavo,* 3, 131, 1965.

17. Edgerton, V.R. and Simpson, D.R., The intermediate muscle fiber of rats and guinea pigs, *J. Histochem. Cytochem.*, 17, 828, 1969.

18. Peter, J.B., Barnard, R., Edgerton, V.R., Gillespie, C.A., and Stempel, K.E., Metabolic profiles of three fiber types of guinea pigs and rabbits, *Biochemistry*, 11, 2627, 1972.

19. Alexander, K.M. and George, J.C., Fibre type composition of the breast muscle of the North American little brown bat and of the Indian giant fruit bat, *J. Anim. Morphol. Physiol.*, 29, 98, 1982.

20. Talesara, C.L. and Kiran, S., Cytophysiology of vertebrate skeletal muscle fibres, *Indian J. Exp. Biol.*, 24, 331, 1986.

21. Hamalainen, N. and Pette, D., The histochemical profiles of fast fiber types IIB, IID, and IIA in skeletal muscles of mouse, rat and rabbit, *J. Histochem. Cytochem.*, 41, 733, 1993.

22. Essén-Gustavsson, B., Activity and inactivity related muscle adaptation in the animal kingdom, in Saltin B., Ed., *Biochemistry of Exercise,* Vol. VI, Human Kinetics Publishers, Champaign, IL, 1984, 435.

23. Pösö, A.R., Nieminen, M., Raulio, J., Räsänen, L.A., and Soveri, T., Skeletal muscle characteristics of racing reindeer (*Rangifer tarandus*), *Comp. Biochem. Physiol.*, 114A, 277, 1996.

24. Rosser, B.W.C. and George, J.C., The avian pectoralis: histochemical characterization and distribution of muscle fiber types, *Can. J. Zool.*, 64, 1174, 1986.

25. Rosser, B.W.C., Wick, M., Waldbillig, D.M., and Bandman, E., Heterogeneity of myosin heavy-chain expression in fast-twitch fiber types of mature avian pectoralis muscle, *Biochem. Cell Biol.*, 74, 715, 1996.

26. Rosser, B.W.C. and George, J.C., Histochemical characterization and distribution of fiber types in the pectoralis muscle of the ostrich (*Struthio camelus*) and emu (*Dromaius novaehollandiae*), *Acta Zool.*, 66, 191, 1985.

27. Buller, A.J., Eccles, J.C., and Eccles, R.M., Interactions between motorneurones and muscles in respect of the characteristic speeds of their responses, *J. Physiol. (London)*, 150, 417, 1960.

28. Golisch, G., Pette, D., and Pichlmaier, H., Metabolic differentiation of rabbit skeletal muscle as induced by specific innervation, *Eur. J. Biochem.*, 16, 110, 1970.

29. Vrbova, G., Influence of activity of some characteristic properties of slow and fast mammalian muscles, in Hutton, R.S. and Miller, D.I., Eds., *Exercise and Sport Sciences Reviews*, Franklin Institute Press, New York, 1977, 181.

30. Edgerton, V.R., Mammalian muscle fiber types and their adaptability, *Am. Zool.*, 18, 113, 1978.

31. Gunn, H.M., The mean fiber area of the semitendinosus, diaphragm and pectoralis transversus muscles in differing types of horse and dog, *J. Anat.*, 127, 403, 1978.

32. Reiter, R.J., Melatonin: the chemical expression of darkness, *Molec. Cell. Endocrinol.*, 79, C153, 1991.

33. Klein, D.C., The pineal gland: a model of neuroendocrine regulation, in Reichlin, S., Baldessarini, R.J., and Martin, J.B., Eds., *The Hypothalamus,* Raven Press, New York, 1978, 303.

34. Klein, D.C. and Moor, R.J., Pineal *N*-acetyltransferase and hydroxyindole-*O*-methyltransferase: control by the retinohypothalamic tract and the suprachiasmatic nucleus, *Brain Res.*, 174, 245, 1978.

35. Ebadi, M., Regulation of the synthesis of melatonin and its significance to neuroendocrinology, in Reiter, R.J., Ed., *The Pineal Gland*, Raven Press, New York, 1984, 1.

36. Gaston, S. and Menaker, M., Pineal function: the biological clock in the sparrow?, *Science*, 160, 1125, 1968.

37. Zimmerman, N. and Menaker, M., The pineal gland: a pacemaker within the circadian system of the house sparrow, *Proc. Natl. Acad. Sci. USA*, 76, 999, 1979.

38. Binkley, S., Kluth, S., and Menaker, M., Pineal function in sparrows: circadian rhythms and body temperature, *Science*, 174, 311, 1971.

39. Binkley, S., Pineal and melatonin: circadian rhythms and body temperature, in Scheving, L., Halberg, F., and Pauly, J., Eds., *Chronobiology*, Igaku Shoin, Tokyo, 1974, 582.

40. Binkley, S., Functions of the pineal gland, in Epple, A. and Stetson, M.H., Eds., *Avian Endocrinology*, Academic Press, New York, 1980, 53.

41. Binkley, S., *The Pineal: Endocrine and Neuroendocrine Function.*, Prentice Hall, Englewood Cliffs, NJ, 1988.

42. McMillan, J.P., Pinealectomy abolishes circadian rhythm of migratory restlessness, *J. Comp. Physiol.*, 79, 105, 1972.

43. Gwinner, E., Effects of pinealectomy on circadian locomotor activity rhythms in European starling, *Sturnus vulgaris, J. Comp. Physiol.*, 126, 123, 1978.

44. Ebihara, S. and Kawamura, H., The role of the pineal and the suprachiasmatic nucleus in the control of circadian locomotor activity rhythms in the Java sparrow, *Padda oryzivora, J. Comp. Physiol.*, 141, 207, 1981.

45. Fuchs, J., Effects of pinealectomy and subsequent melatonin implants on activity rhythms in the house finch (*Carpodacus mexicanus*), *J. Comp. Physiol.*, 153, 413, 1983.

46. Simpson, S.M. and Follett, B.F., Pineal and hypothalamic pacemakers: their role in regulating circadian rhythmicity in Japanese quail, *J. Comp. Physiol.*, 144, 381, 1981.

47. Ebihara, S., Uchiyama, K., and Oshima, I., Circadian organization in the pigeon, *Columba livia*: the role of the pineal organ and the eye, *J. Comp. Physiol.*, A154, 59, 1984.

48. Foa, A. and Menaker, M., Contribution of pineal and retinae to the circadian rhythms of circulating melatonin in pigeons, *J. Comp. Physiol.*, A164, 25, 1988.

49. Oshima, I., Yamada, H., Goto, M., Sato, K., and Ebihara, S., Pineal and retinal melatonin is involved in the control of circadian locomotor activity and body temperature rhythms in the pigeon, *J. Comp. Physiol.*, A166, 217, 1989.

50. Underwood, H. and Menaker, M., Extraretinal light perception: entrainment of the biological clock controlling lizard locomotor activity, *Science*, 170, 190, 1970.

51. Quay, W.B., Individuation and lack of pineal effect in the rat's circardian locomotor rhythm, *Physiol. Behav.*, 3, 109, 1968.

52. Roth, J.J., Gern, W.A., Roth, E.C., Ralph, C.L., and Jacobson, E., Nonpineal melatonin in the alligator (*Alligator mississippiensis*), *Science*, 210, 548, 1980.

53. Harlow, H.J., Phillips, J.A., and Ralph, C.L., Day-night rhythm in plasma melatonin in a mammal lacking a distinct pineal gland, the nine-banded armadillo, *Gen. Comp. Endocrinol.*, 45, 212, 1981.

54. Wetterberg, L., Melatonin in humans: physiological and clinical studies, *J. Neural Trans. Suppl.*, 13, 282, 1978.

55. Arendt, J. and Broadway, J., Light and melatonin as zeitgebers in man, *Chronobiol. Int.*, 4, 273, 1987.

56. Arendt, J., Aldhous, M., and Wright, J. Synchronization of a disturbed sleep-wave cycle in a blind man by melatonin, *Lancet*, 1, 772, 1988.

57. Petterborg, L.J., Thalén, B.-E., Kjellman, B.F., and Wetterberg, L., Effect of melatonin replacement on serum hormone rhythms in a patient lacking endogenous melatonin, *Brain Res. Bull.*, 27, 181, 1991.

58. Bartness, T.J. and Goldman, B.D., Mammalian pineal melatonin: a clock for all seasons, *Experientia*, 45, 936, 1989.

59. Osei, P., Robbins, K.R., and Shirley, H.V., Effects of exogenous melatonin on growth and energy metabolism in chickens, *Nutr. Res.*, 9, 69, 1989.

60. Zeman, M., Vyboh, P., Jurani, M., Lamosova, D., Kostal, L., Bolcik, B., Blazicek, P., and Juraniova, E., Effects of exogenous melatonin on some endocrine, behavioural and metabolic parameters in Japanese quail *Coturnix coturnix japonica*, *Comp. Biochem. Physiol.*, 105A, 323, 1993.

61. John, T.M. and George, J.C., Seasonal ultrastructural changes in the pineal gland of the migratory Canada goose, *Cytobios*, 58, 179, 1989.

62. George, J.C., Physiological adaptations in the rosy pastor wintering in India, in Ripley, II, S.D., Ed., *A Bundle of Feathers*, Oxford University Press, Delhi, 1978, 49.

63. McKeown, B.A., John, T.M., and George, J.C., Diurnal variation in effects of melatonin on plasma growth hormone and glucose in the pigeon, *Endocrinol. Exp.*, 9, 263, 1975.

64. Darre, M.J., Cogburn, L.A., and Harrison, P.C., The effect of pinealectomy on the metabolism and somatic growth of immature cockerels, *Poultry Sci.*, 59, 2574, 1980.

65. John, T.M., Viswanathan, M., George, J.C., and Scanes, C.G., Influence of chronic melatonin implantation on circulating levels of catecholamines, growth hormone, thyroid hormones, glucose, and free fatty acids in the pigeon, *Gen. Comp. Endocrinol.*, 79, 226, 1990.

66. Vriend, J., Sheppard, M.S., and Borer, K.T., Melatonin increases serum growth hormone and insulin-like growth factor I (IGF-I) levels in male Syrian hamsters via hypothamic neurotransmitters, *Growth, Development and Aging*, 54, 165, 1990.

67. Reiter, R.J., The melatonin rhythm: both a clock and a calendar, *Experientia*, 49, 654, 1993.

68. John, T.M., Itoh, S., and George, J.C., On the role of the pineal in thermoregulation in the pigeon, *Hormone Res.*, 9, 41, 1978.

69. George, J.C., Thermogenesis in the avian body and the role of the pineal in thermoregulation, in Reiter, R.J., Ed., *The Pineal and Its Hormones*, Alan R. Liss, New York, 1982, 217.

70. Balsam, A., Dobbs, C.R., and Leppo, L.E., Circadian variations in concentrations of plasma thyroxine and triiodothyronine in man, *J. Appl. Physiol.*, 39, 297, 1975.

71. John, T.M. and George, J.C., Diurnal thermal response to pinealectomy and photoperiod in the pigeon, *J. Interdiscipl. Cycle Res.*, 15, 57, 1984.

72. Steen, J. and Steen, J.B., The importance of the legs in the thermoregulation of birds, *Acta Physiol. Scand.*, 63, 285, 1965.

73. Baudinette, R.V., Loveridge, J.F., Mills, C.P., Schmidt-Nielsen, K., and Wilson, K.J., Heat loss from feet of Herring Gulls at rest and during flight, *Am. J. Physiol.*, 230, 920, 1976.

74. Bernstein, M.H., Vascular responses and foot temperature in pigeons, *Am. J. Physiol.*, 226, 1350, 1974.

75. George, J.C., Thermogenesis in birds, in Hales, J.R.S., Ed., *Thermal Physiology*, Raven Press, New York, 1984, 467.

76. George, J.C. and John, T.M., Physiological responses to cold exposure in pigeons, in Heller, H.C., Musacchia, X.J., and Wang, L.C.H., Eds., *Living in the Cold*, Elsevier, New York, 1986, 435.

77. Viswanathan, M., Hissa, R., and George, J.C., Suppression of sympathetic nervous system by short photoperiod and melatonin in the Syrian hamster, *Life Sci.*, 38, 73, 1986.

78. Viswanathan, M., Hissa, R., and George, J.C., Effects of short photoperiod and melatonin treatment on thermogenesis in the Syrian hamster, *J. Pineal Res.*, 3, 311, 1986.

79. Lee, P.N., Allen, A.E., and Pang, S.F., Cold stress during scotophase elicited differential responses in quail pineal, retinal, and serum melatonin levels, *Acta Endocrinol.*, 122, 535, 1990.

80. George, J.C., Thermoregulatory and metabolic responses to cold exposure in birds, in Maitra, S.K., Ed., *Frontiers in Environmental and Metabolic Endocrinology*, University of Burdwan, India, 1997, 135.

81. Raman, E.R., Roberts, M.F., and Vanhuyse, V.J., Body temperature control of rat tail blood flow, *Am. J. Physiol.*, 245, R426, 1983.

82. Arutyunyan, G.S., Mashkovskii, M.D., and Roschina, L.F., Pharmacological properties of melatonin, *Fed. Proc. Fed. Am. Soc. Exp. Biol.*, 23, T1330, 1964.

83. Barchas, J.D., DaCosta, F., and Spector, S., Acute pharmacology of melatonin, *Nature*, 214, 919, 1967.

84. Fioretti, M.C., Riccardi, C., Menconi, E., and Martini, L., Control of the circadian rhythm of the body temperature in the rat, *Life Sci.*, 14, 211, 1974.

85. Lynch, G.R., White, S.E., Grundel, R., and Berger, M.S., Effects of photoperiod, melatonin administration and thyroid block on spontaneous daily torpor and temperature regulation in the white-footed mouse, *Peromyscus leucopus*, *J. Comp. Physiol.*, 125, 157, 1978.

86. Palmer, D.L. and Riedesel, M.L., Responses of whole-animal and isolated hearts of ground squirrels, *Citellus lateralis*, to melatonin, *Comp. Biochem. Physiol.*, 53C, 69, 1976.

87. Smith, R.E. and Horwitz, B.A., Brown fat and thermogenesis, *Physiol. Rev.*, 49, 330, 1969.

88. Foster, D.O. and Frydman, M.L., Tissue distribution of cold-induced thermogenesis in conscious warm- and cold-acclimated rats reevaluated from changes in tissue blood flow: the dominant role of brown adipose tissue in the replacement of shivering by non-shivering thermogenesis, *Can. J. Physiol. Pharmacol.*, 57, 257, 1979.

89. Heldmaier, G.K. and Hoffman, K., Melatonin stimulates growth of brown adipose tissue, *Nature*, 247, 224, 1974.

90. Reiter, R.J., Changes in pituitary prolactin levels of female hamsters as a function of age, photoperiod and pinealectomy, *Acta Endocrinol.*, 79, 43, 1975.

91. Viswanathan, M. and George, J.C., Pinealectomy has no effect on diet-induced thermogenesis and brown adipose tissue proliferation in rats, *J. Pineal Res.*, 1, 69, 1984.

92. Kavaliers, M., Peptides, the pineal gland and thermoregulation, in Reiter, R.J., Ed., *The Pineal and Its Hormones*, Alan R. Liss, New York, 1982, 207.

93. Kasbohn, P., Der Einfluss des Lichtes auf die Temperaturadaptation bei *Rana temporaria, Helgolander Wissensch. Meersuntersuchungen*, 16, 157, 1967.

94. Hutchison, V.H. and Kosh, R.J., Thermoregulatory function of the parietal eye in the lizard *Anolis carolinensis, Oecologia*, 16, 173, 1974.

95. Ralph, C.L., Firth, B.T., Gern, W.A., and Owens, D.W., The pineal complex and thermoregulation, *Biol. Rev.*, 54, 41, 1979.

96. Ralph, C.L., Pineal bodies and thermoregulation, in Reiter, R.J., Ed., *The Pineal Gland*, Raven Press, New York, 1984, 193.

97. Saarela, S. and Reiter, R.J., Function of melatonin in thermoregulatory processes, *Life Sci.*, 54, 295, 1994.

98. Strassman, R.J., Qualls, C.R., Lisansky, E.J., and Peake, G.T., Elevated rectal temperature produced by all-night bright light is reversed by melatonin infusion in man, *J. Appl. Physiol.*, 71, 2178, 1991.

99. Vakkuri, O., Lamsa, E., Rahkamaa, E., Ruotsalainen, H., and Leppaluoto, J., Iodinated melatonin: preparation and characterization of the molecular structure by mass and ¹HNMR spectroscopy, *Analyt. Biochem.*, 142, 284, 1984.

100. Vanecek, J., Pavlik, A., and Illnerova, H., Hypothalamic melatonin receptor sites revealed by autoradiography, *Brain Res.*, 435, 359, 1987.

101. Baker, M.A., A brain-cooling system in mammals, *Sci. Am.*, 240, 130, 1979.

102. Young, A.A. and Dawson, N.J., Evidence for on-off control of heat dissipation from the tail of the rat, *Can. J. Physiol. Pharmacol.*, 60, 392, 1982.

103. Viswanathan, M., Laitinen, J.T., and Saavedra, J.M., Expression of melatonin receptors in arteries involved in thermoregulation, *Proc. Natl. Acad. Sci. USA*, 87, 6200, 1990.

104. Evans, B.K., Mason, R., and Wilson, V.G., Evidence for direct vasoconstrictor activity of melatonin in pressurized segments of isolated caudal artery from juvenile rats, *Naunyn-Schmiedeberg's Arch. Pharmacol.*, 346, 362, 1992.

105. Laitinen, J.T., Viswanathan, M., Vakkuri, O., and Saavedra, J.M., Differential regulation of rat melatonin receptors: selective age-associated decline and lack of melatonin-induced changes, *Endocrinology*, 130, 2139, 1992.

106. Viswanathan, M., Laitenen, J.T., and Saavedra, J.M., Vascular melatonin receptors, *Biol. Signals*, 2, 221, 1993.

107. Sugden, D., Melatonin: binding site characteristics and biochemical and cellular responses, *Neurochem. Int.*, 24, 147, 1994.

108. John, T.M. and George, J.C., Physiological responses of melatonin-implanted pigeons to changes in ambient temperature, in Riklis, E., Ed., *Photobiology*, Plenum Press, New York, 1991, 597.

109. Hissa, R., George, J.C., and Saarela, S., Dose-related effects of noradrenaline and corticosterone on temperature regulation in the pigeon, *Comp. Biochem. Physiol.*, 65C, 25, 1980.

110. Weekley, L.B., Melatonin-induced relaxation of rat aorta: interaction with adrenergic agonists, *J. Pineal Res.*, 11, 28, 1991.

111. Hardeland, R., The presence and function of melatonin and structurally related indoleamines in a dinoflagellate, and a hypothesis on the evolutionary significance of these tryptophan metabolites in unicellulars, *Experientia*, 49, 614, 1993.

112. Hardeland, R. and Fuhrberg, B., Ubiquitous melatonin-presence and effects in unicells, plants and animals, *Trends Comp. Biochem. Physiol.*, 2, 25, 1996.

113. Ebadi, M., Samejima, M., and Pfeiffer, R.F., Pineal gland synchronizing and refining physiological events, *News Physiol. Sci.*, 8, 30, 1993.

114. Hardeland, R., Poeggeler, B., Balzer, I., and Behrmann, G., A hypothesis on the evolutionary origins of photoperiodism based on circadian rhythmicity of melatonin in phylogenetically distant organisms, in Gutenbrunner, C., Hildebrandt, G., and Moog, R., Eds., *Chronobiology and Chronomedicine*, Peter Lang, Verlag, 1993, 113.

115. Csaba, G., Presence in and effects of pineal indoleamines at very low level of phylogeny, *Experientia*, 49, 627, 1993.

116. Vivien-Roels, B. and Pévet, P., Melatonin: presence and formation in invertebrates, *Experientia*, 49, 642, 1993.

117. Reiter, R.J., Poeggeler, B., Tan, D.-X., Chen, L.-D., Manchester, L.C., and Guerrero, J.M., Antioxidant capacity of melatonin: a novel action not requiring a receptor, *Neuroendocrinol. Lett.*, 15, 103, 1993.

118. Huether, G., The contribution of extrapineal sites of melatonin synthesis to circulating melatonin levels in higher vertebrates, *Experientia*, 49, 665, 1993.

119. John, T.M. and George, J.C., Physiological responses to vagotomized pigeons exposed to ambient temperatures gradually reduced from 34°C to 2°C, *J. Auton. Nerv. Syst.*, 18, 153, 1987.

120. Zisapel, N., Melatonin receptors revisited, *J. Neural Transm.*, 73, 1, 1988.

121. Cunnane, S.C., Manku, M., Oka, M., and Horralein, D.F., Enhanced vascular reactivity to various constrictor agents following pinealectomy in the rat: role of melatonin, *Can. J. Physiol. Pharmacol.*, 58, 287, 1980.

122. Newsholme, E. and Leech, T., *The Runner*, W.L. Meagher, Fitness Books, NJ, 1985.

123. John, T.M. and George, J.C., Diurnal variation in the effect of melatonin on plasma and muscle free fatty acid levels in the pigeon, *Endocrinol. Exp.*, 10, 131, 1976.

124. John, T.M., George, J.C., and Brown, G.M., Effect of exercise by *in vivo* electrical stimulation of the pectoral muscles on daytime blood melatonin levels in the pigeon, *Cytobios*, 72, 167, 1992.

125. John, T.M., George, J.C., Yie, S.M., and Brown, G.M., Flight-induced increase in circulatory levels of melatonin in the homing pigeon, *Comp. Biochem. Physiol.*, 106A, 645, 1993.

126. Sandyk, R., and Kay, S.R., Melatonin as a mediator of atypical antipsychotic drug effects, *Schizophrenia Res.*, 4, 59, 1991.

127. Aulie, A., Body temperatures in pigeons and budgerigars during sustained flight, *Comp. Biochem. Physiol.*, 39A, 173, 1971.

128. Strassman, R.J., Appenzeller, O., Lewy, A.J., Qualls, C.R., and Peake, G.T., Increase
      in plasma melatonin, β-endorphin, and cortisol after a 28.5-mile mountain race:
      relationship to performance and lack of effect of naltrexone., *J. Clin. Endocrinol.
      Metab.*, 69, 540, 1989.

129. Fernstrom, J.D. and Wurtman, R.J., Nutrition and the brain, *Sci. Am.*, 230, 84, 1974.

130. Reiter, R.J., Pineal melatonin: cell biology of its synthesis and of its physiological
      interactions, *Endocr. Rev.*, 12, 151, 1991.

131. Farrell, P.A., Gates, W.K., Maksud, M.G., and Morgan, W.P., Increases in plasma β-
      endorphin/β-lipotropin immunoreactivity after treadmill running in humans, *J. Appl.
      Physiol.*, 52, 1245, 1982.

132. Viswanathan, M., van Dijk, J.P., Graham, T.E., Bonen, A., and George, J.C., Exer-
      cise- and cold-induced changes in plasma β-endorphin and β-lipotropin in men and
      women, *J. Appl. Physiol.*, 62, 622, 1987.

133. John, T.M., Viswanathan, M., and George, J.C., Immunocytochemical localization
      and seasonal changes in staining intensity of β-endorphin-like immunoreactivity in
      the adenohypophysis of the migratory Canada goose, *Cytobios*, 56, 179, 1988.

134. Hikida, R.S., Staron, R.S., Hagerman, F.C., Sharman, W.M., and Costill, D.L., Muscle
      fiber necrosis associated with human marathon runners, *J. Neurol. Sci.*, 59, 185, 1983.

135. George, J.C., John, T.M., and Minhas, K.J., Seasonal degenerative, reparative and
      regenerative ultrastructural changes in the breast muscle of the migratory Canada
      goose, *Cytobios*, 52, 109, 1987.

136. Grinyer, I. and George, J.C., Some observations on the ultrastructure of the humming-
      bird pectoral muscles, *Can. J. Zool.*, 47, 771, 1969.

137. Poeggeler, B., Reiter, R.J., Tan, D.-X., Chen, L.-D., and Manchester, L.C., Melatonin,
      hydroxyl radical-mediated oxidative damage, and aging: a hypothesis, *J. Pineal Res.*,
      14, 151, 1993.

138. George, J.C. and John, T.M., Flight effects on certain blood parameters in homing
      pigeons, *Columba livia, Comp. Biochem. Physiol.*, 106A, 707, 1993.

139. George, J.C., Physiological significance of flight-induced changes in certain hor-
      monal, metabolite and other blood values in homing pigeons, in Joy, K.P., Krishna,
      A., and Halder, C., Eds., *Comparative Endocrinology and Reproduction*, Narosa
      Publishing House, New Delhi, 1997, p. 602.

140. Vaughan, G.M., Melatonin in humans, in Reiter, R.J., Ed., *Pineal Research Reviews*,
      II, Alan R. Liss, New York, 1984, 141.

141. Haase, E., Rees, A., and Harvey, S., Flight stimulates adrenocortical activity in
      pigeons (*Columba livia*), *Gen. Comp. Endocrinol.*, 61, 424, 1986.

142. Viswanathan, M., John, T.M., George, J.C., and Etches, R.J., Flight effects on plasma
      glucose, lactate, catecholamines and corticosterone in homing pigeons, *Horm. Metabol.
      Res.*, 19, 400, 1987.

143. Carr, D.B., Reppert, S.M., Bullen, B.A., Skrinar, G.S., Beitins, I.Z., Arnold, M.A.,
      Rosenblatt, M., Martin, J.B., and McArthur, J.W., Plasma melatonin increases during
      exercise in women, *J. Clin. Endocrinol. Metab.*, 53, 224, 1981.

144. Ronkainen, H., Vakkuri, O., and Kauppila, A., Effects of physical exercise on the serum concentration of melatonin in female runners, *Acta Obstet. Gynecol. Scand.*, 65, 827, 1986.

145. Berga, S.L., Mortola, J.F., and Yen, S.S.C., Amplification of nocturnal melatonin secretion in women with functional hypothalamic amenorrhea, *J. Clin. Endocrinol. Metab.*, 66, 242, 1988.

146. Glass, J.D. and Knotts, L.K., A brain site for the antigonadal action of melatonin in the white-footed mouse (*Peromyscus leucopus*): involvement of the immunoreactive GnRH neuronal system, *Neuroendocrinology*, 46, 48, 1987.

147. Vanecek, J. and Klein, D.C., Melatonin inhibits gonadotropin-releasing hormone-induced elevation of intracellular Ca^{2+} in neonatal rat pituitary cells, *Endocrinology*, 130, 701, 1992.

148. Laatikainen, T., Virtanen, T., and Apter, D., Plasma immunoreactive β-endorphin in exercise-associated amenorrhea, *Am. J. Obstet. Gynecol.*, 154, 94, 1986.

149. Vanecek, J., Mechanism of melatonin action, *Physiol. Res.*, 40, 11, 1991.

150. Graham, T.E., Viswanathan, M., van Dijk, J.P., Bonen, A., and George, J.C., Thermal and metabolic responses to cold by men and by eumenorrheic and amenorrheic women, *J. Appl. Physiol.*, 67, 282, 1989.

151. Tolis, G. and Diamanti, E., Distress amenorrhea, *Ann. N.Y. Acad. Sci.*, 771, 660, 1995.

Chapter 6

Melatonin-Kidney Interactions

Yong Song, Gregory M. Brown,
Shiu-Fun Pang, and Mel Silverman

Contents

Introduction

First described by Galen (130–200 A.D.), the pineal gland was once considered as the "seat of the soul". Its detailed anatomical localization was described by Plater (1583), Bauhin (1590), Harvey (1616), and Riolan (1626).[1] In the late 19th century, it was speculated that in lower vertebrates the pineal gland acted as a "third eye" (Rabl-Ruckhard, 1882; Ahlborn, 1883; de Graaf, 1886).[1] Despite the fact that, in 1917, McCord and Allen[2] reported that pineal extracts induced dramatic lightening

0-8493-8564-4/99/$0.00+$.50
© 1999 by CRC Press LLC

of frog skin, there was little followup to this observation. Further progress did not occur until the biochemical isolation of melatonin from pineal extracts[3] and determination of its structure.[4]

One of the major breakthroughs in pineal research occurred when it was demonstrated that the pineal gland participates in the regulation of diurnal rhythms.[5,6] Diurnal activity of the pineal gland itself is mediated by sympathetic nervous system response to light entering through the eyes.[7,8] The synthesis and release of pineal melatonin exhibit a circadian rhythm resulting in low plasma melatonin concentrations during daylight hours and peak concentrations at night (dark phase).[9-11] Seasonal changes of melatonin concentration in the pineal gland and plasma are associated with the natural light/dark cycle.[9-11]

Although it has been recognized for some time that the pineal gland plays an important role in reproductive biology in different species,[12,13] only recently has it become apparent that melatonin plays a role in modulating a wide variety of nonendocrine as well as endocrine functions,[11,14] including the immune,[15-17] excretory,[18,19] and cardiovascular systems,[20] as well as thermoregulation.[21-23] Melatonin also interacts specifically with kidney,[24] adrenals,[25-27] thyroid,[28,29] and intestine.[30,31]

The main thrust of this chapter is to focus on renal regulatory effects of melatonin, but before elaborating on potential functional melatonin-kidney interactions, it is necessary to review briefly the modern concepts of the cellular action of melatonin.

Molecular Mechanism of Melatonin Action

A major breakthrough in melatonin research occurred with the synthesis of 2-[^{125}I]iodomelatonin. The availability of this radioligand made it possible to identify and quantitate specific melatonin receptors (MR), permitting determination of MR organ distribution and their pharmacokinetic characterization.[32-35] The presence in tissues of specific high-affinity MR has strong biologic implications, suggesting that the cellular action of melatonin is effected through membrane transduction and intracellular signaling following melatonin binding to its receptor.

The next milestone was the cloning of MR in different species.[36-40] From the sequence information obtained, it was established that MR belong to the family of G-coupled, seven-transmembrane receptors. So far, two mammalian subtypes of high-affinity melatonin receptors have been identified, Mel-1a[37] and Mel-1b.[38] However, except for differences in their predicted amino acid sequence, there is no experimental evidence to indicate any significant functional variation of these two MR subtypes.

Investigation of the mechanism of MR activation, primarily using cells of neural origin, has demonstrated that both MR subtypes are regulated by a pertussis toxin-sensitive G-protein (G_i). Thus, binding of melatonin to Mel-1a or Mel-1b leads to activation of G_i which in turn inhibits the activity of adenyl cyclase, resulting in a decrease of the intracellular second messenger, cAMP.[37-39] This scheme is illustrated in Figure 1.

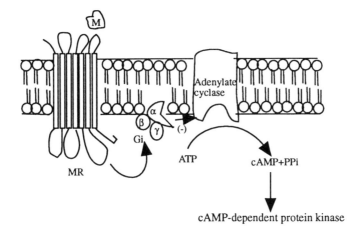

FIGURE 1
Signaling cascade of MR after the activation of its ligand, melatonin (M); (−) indicates inhibitory effect.

Melatonin Effects on the Kidney

Physiological Studies

In the 1960s and 1970s, the results of *in vivo* studies suggested that melatonin might play a renal regulatory role, affecting urine output and cation excretion,[18,42–45] but there was some inconsistency in these early findings. Later reports indicated that the renal effects of melatonin might be species specific.[19,46] In nocturnal animals, such as hamsters, melatonin administration induces an increase in urine output.[19] In contrast, melatonin infusion causes a reduction in the glomerular filtration rate in diurnal animals, such as ewes.[46]

There is also experimental evidence indicating a relationship between melatonin blood levels and urine cation excretion. For example: (1) prior to the biochemical isolation of melatonin from the pineal gland, it had been found that administration of pineal extract induced strong sodium retention;[44] (2) reduction in sodium and potassium excretion was also recorded in pinealectomized rats;[18] (3) decreases in sodium and potassium concentration and urine osmolality were observed following melatonin administration to hamsters;[19] and (4) alterations of plasma melatonin levels are associated with changes in plasma concentration of other ions, such as calcium, magnesium, and zinc.[45,47,48]

In man, there is a normally observed nocturnal decrease in urine volume and an approximate 50% decrease in excretion rate of sodium, potassium, chloride, and urate. These changes correlate with the peak plasma concentration of melatonin.[49,50] In contrast, phosphate reabsorption decreases during the day, when the plasma melatonin level is low.[51]

Mechanistically, it was initially uncertain whether the renal effects of melatonin were secondary to some hemodynamic or other systemic (hormonal) changes caused

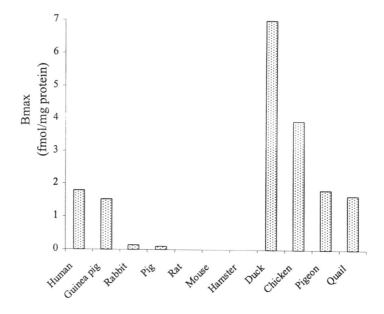

FIGURE 2

Maximum binding densities (B_{max}) of renal 2-[^{125}I]iodomelatonin binding sites in various species. Results are means of 3 to 8 tests.

by melatonin or whether they were due to a direct action of melatonin on kidney tissue. As discussed in greater detail below, a substantial body of evidence, accumulated over the last few years, has demonstrated that MR are localized in kidney tissue.[24,52–57] This finding is highly suggestive of a direct renal functional role for melatonin.

In the remainder of this chapter we will review new data implicating melatonin in the regulation of kidney function. Although the physiologic evidence described above suggests that melatonin might have both glomerular as well as tubular actions, the weight of the experimental information to be presented will focus on the renal epithelial effects.

Characterization of MR Using Radioligand Binding

Quantitation of MR in kidney tissue of different species has been carried out by means of 2-[^{125}I]iodomelatonin binding studies. As shown in Figure 2, specific MR are expressed in the kidney of man,[54] guinea pig,[24,53] pig, rabbit, duck, chicken, pigeon, and quail.[56] There are no detectable MR in the kidney of rat and mouse, and the expression level of MR in avian kidney is greater than that found in mammals. Ontogenic studies show that MR are found in embryonic kidney of chickens,[58] guinea pigs,[59] and humans;[57] are expressed at higher levels in young animals; and decline with age (Figure 3).[58,59]

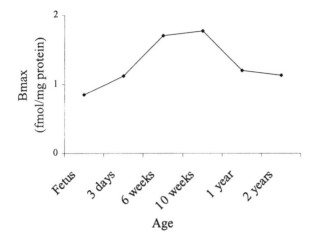

FIGURE 3

Developmental changes of B_{max} of 2-[^{125}I]iodomelatonin binding sites in the guinea pig kidney. Data are means of five samples.

In all species, MR are of high affinity, with an equilibrium dissociation constant (K_d) of 20 to 60 pM, and exhibit pharmacologic specificity for melatonin and its analogues.[52-54,56] Further, based on autoradiographic studies of guinea pig kidney, MR are localized mainly in the cortex.[53]

Molecular Characterization of Renal MR

Using primers specific for Mel-1a or Mel-1b, we attempted to detect Mel-1a and Mel-1b by polymerase chain reaction (PCR) from a commercially available human kidney cDNA library (derived from an adult male, Gibco BRL) as well as from primary cultures of human kidney epithelia cells. As indicated in Figure 4, we found that after 30 cycles only Mel-1a, but not Mel-1b, could be detected by ethidium bromide staining of the agarose gel. However, after 50 cycles of PCR, a very weak Mel-1b band became visible (data not shown). It is important to note that in the experiment depicted in Figure 4, the reagents used for PCR were identical for Mel-1a and Mel-1b, except for the use of different primers. Also, as a control, we confirmed that when equal amounts of cloned Mel-1a and Mel-1b in plasmid were used as templates, the Mel-1a and Mel-1b PCR products obtained were equal (Song and Silverman, unpublished observation),[60] thus verifying that the primers selected for Mel-1a and Mel-1b were capable of amplifying Mel-1a or Mel-1b with similar efficiency in PCR. For these reasons, we have concluded that a majority of MR in human kidney as well as in primary cultures of human renal epithelial cells are of the Mel-1a subtype. Although Mel-1b is also expressed, it is present at a much lower level. In a cell line derived from human embryonic kidney (HEK293)[60,62] and in human fetal kidney,[57] similar results have been reported using PCR[60,62] or by *in situ* hybridization.[57]

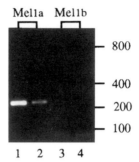

FIGURE 4
PCR of Mel-1a (lanes 1 and 2) and Mel-1b (lanes 3 and 4) from human kidney cDNA library (lanes 1 and 3) and reverse transcription product of total RNA from primary culture human renal cortical epithelia cells (lanes 2 and 4). Primers for Mel-1a and Mel-1b are as reported.[37,60] Molecular size marker (bp) is indicated. Total RNA was extracted and reverse transcription was performed as reported.[60] PCR was performed for 30 cycles at 94°C for 30 sec, 58°C for 30 sec, and 72°C for 30 sec. The resulting PCR products were subjected to 1.5% agarose gel and staining by ethidium bromide. The PCR products had been confirmed by sequencing.

In chickens, it has been reported that Mel-1b is expressed in the kidney as detected by northern blot analysis,[40] but there is no report regarding Mel-1a or Mel-1c expression in either chicken or avian kidney.

So far, there has been no report of any functional difference between Mel-1a and Mel-1b. Whether there is any physiological implication of the observed difference in expression of Mel-1a and Mel-1b in the kidney remains to be determined.

The presence of kidney MR as established by radioligand binding studies and mRNA expression is suggestive but is only indirect evidence of a melatonin-renal functional linkage. To gain further insight as to the possible nature of a renal physiologic role for melatonin we sought to determine (1) the intrarenal cellular localization of MR, and (2) whether there is evidence that melatonin interaction with renal MR gives rise to cellular changes in biologic activity.

Localization of MR in Guinea Pig Kidney

Using a peptide specific polyclonal antibody against Mel-1a, we have found that Mel-1a is expressed mainly at the basolateral membrane (BLM) of cortical epithelial cells in guinea pig kidney (Figure 5).[26] Moreover, pharmacologic characterization of MR in a cortical BLM fraction enriched in Na-K-ATPase activity demonstrates that these cortical BLM MR exhibit high affinity (Figure 6) and a pharmacolgic specificity profile specific for melatonin and its analogs.[24] Finally, as shown in Figure 5, the native form of renal BLM Mel-1a is expressed as a 37-kDa protein on western blots, the same as detected in human and rat brain.[24]

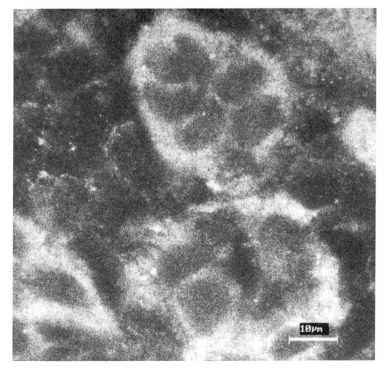

FIGURE 5
Immunolabeling of Mel-1a in the guinea pig proximal tubules by a peptide specific antibody against Mel-1a indicates predominant basolateral membrane labeling. (From Song, Y. et al., *FASEB J.*, 11, 93, 1997. With permission.)

Biologic Activity of Renal MR

Renal MR Are G_i Coupled

2-[^{125}I]Iodomelatonin binding in human,[54] guinea pig,[53] and chicken[56] kidney is inhibited by GTPγS, implying that renal MR are coupled to G-proteins. More recently, we have shown that MR in guinea pig renal BLM are coupled to G_i as indicated by the inhibitory effects of GTPγS (Figures 6 and 7) and pertussis toxin on 2-[^{125}I]iodomelatonin binding.[53] In tissue explant sections from chicken kidney, melatonin inhibits forskolin-stimulated cAMP production, and this effect is abolished when Gi is blocked by preincubation with pertussis toxin.

The findings described above, demonstrating that renal BLM MR are G_i coupled are in complete agreement with previous *in vitro* studies showing that cloned Mel-1a[37] and Mel-1b[38] from brain and retina are coupled to G_i and inhibit adenylate cyclase activity in various cell lines.

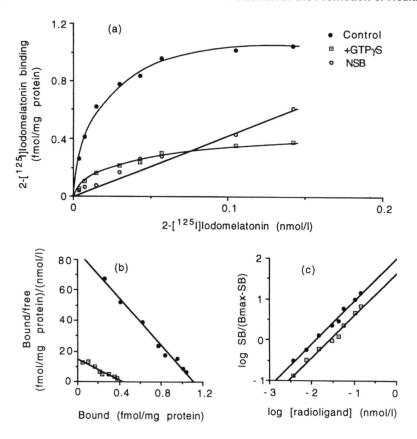

FIGURE 6

Specific 2-[125I]iodomelatonin binding in guinea pig renal BLM. Binding affinity and density of 2-[125I]iodomelatonin in BLM were inhibited by 100 μM GTPγS. (a) Specific and nonspecific binding (NSB) curves. (b) Scatchard plots and Hill plots of specific binding data are shown. (From Song, Y. et al., *FASEB J.*, 11, 93, 1997. With permission.)

Renal MR and Regulation of Cellular Cyclic AMP

The foregoing evidence that renal MR are localized to BLM of cortical epithelial cells, in particular those of the proximal tubule, is highly suggestive that melatonin has a direct effect on renal epithelia. Further, the demonstration that MR are also localized to the BLM of small intestinal cells[24] supports the concept for a generalized action of melatonin on epithelial tissue that may be different than what takes place in the brain.

In order to explore the melatonin-epithelial interaction in greater detail, we sought a suitable *in vitro* system. After assaying a number of epithelial cell lines for the presence of high-affinity MR, we found that HEK 293 cells (determined to be of epithelial origin based on intermediate filament characterization) have a similar binding capacity of 2-[125I]iodomelatonin as does human kidney cortex (1–1.2 fmol/mg

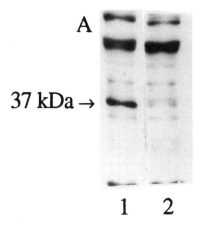

FIGURE 7
Immunoblot analysis of guinea pig renal BLM by a peptide specific antibody of Mel-1a indicates that MR in BLM are expressed as a 37-kDa protein. Lane 2 is a peptide blocked blot. (From Song, Y. et al., *FASEB J.*, 11, 93, 1997. With permission.)

protein).[54,60] Moreover, the inhibitory effects of GTPγS and pertussis toxin on the binding affinity indicated that MR in this cell line are also G_i-coupled receptors. In addition, pertussis toxin blocked the inhibitory action of melatonin on forskolin-stimulated cAMP levels, another demonstration that MR in HEK cells are G_i-coupled (Figure 8). It is important to note that expression of MR in HEK 293 cells decreases

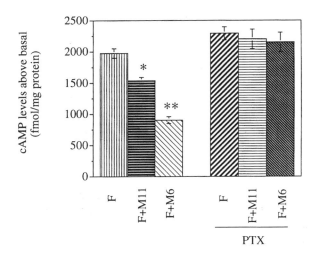

FIGURE 8
Effects of 10 p*M* (M11) or 1 μ*M* (M6) of melatonin on forskolin (10 μ*M*, F) stimulated cAMP level in HEK cells. PTX indicates cells were preincubated 18 hr with 100 ng/ml pertussis toxin. (From Chan, C.W.Y. et al., *Endocrinology*, 188, 4732, 1997. With permission.)

dramaticaly at high passages, and under these conditions there is no detectable 2-[^{125}I]iodomelatonin high-affinity binding (Song and Silverman, unpublished results). For this reason, in our experiments we have only used cells between passage 35 and 55. (This difficulty may account for the recent report by Conway[62] suggesting that melatonin does not interfere with stimulated cAMP levels in HEK cells.)

A logical conclusion from studies using the HEK "model" is that the action of melatonin on epithelial cells, in particular on the renal tubule, may be explained as a nonspecific downregulation of intracellular cAMP. To investigate this issue in more depth, we elected to test whether a melatonin-induced decrease of cAMP was a general phenomenon capable of countering increases in cAMP through occupancy of any G_s-coupled receptor, or whether there was any selectivity involved (i.e., whether there was specific "crosstalk" between G_i-coupled MR and any other G_s-coupled receptors). Accordingly, HEK 293 cells were transiently transfected (separately) with receptors for parathormone, dopamine D1, glucagon-like peptide, and glucose-dependent-insulinotropic peptide. Individually, following transfection, each of the hormones was able to stimulate intracellular cAMP. However, melatonin was only found to decrease intracellular cAMP in the case of the dopamine D1 receptor. It is likely, therefore, that MR and dopamine D1 receptor share the same isozyme of adnylate cyclase.[61]

The HEK 293 cell line may prove useful for more detailed exploration of the cellular and epithelial effects of melatonin, keeping in mind, of course, the dangers inherent in extrapolating from the behavior observed in an *in vitro* cell culture system to the *in vivo* state.

Summary and Conclusion

Our data and those of other investigators indicate that MR are expressed in the kidney of various species. In man, the majority of MR are of Mel-1a subtype. Mel-1b is also expressed in human kidney, but at much lower levels compared to Mel-1a. MR is expressed in cortical epithelial cells and is localized particularly to the basolateral membrane of the proximal tubule. MR in the kidney are coupled to G_i, similar to what has been reported in neural tissues and cloned Mel-1a. Melatonin occupancy of renal MR results in inhibition of adenylate cyclase and a decrease in the intracellular second mesenger cAMP. It is intriguing that melatonin only inhibits certain isoform(s) of adenylate cyclase. Our data showing that MR (Mel-1a) and dopamine D1 interact may have broad implications. One of the hypotheses that needs to be explored is that the effects of melatonin at the cellular level in renal and perhaps neural tissue are mediated by an antidopaminergic action.

Finally, as indicated above, the physiologic actions of melatonin on the kidney can be interpreted as being the result of both glomerular and tubular effects. Much of the experimental evidence discussed in this chapter has focused on melatonin-epithelial interaction(s), presumably underlying the basis for melatonin action on renal tubules. But, the possibility of a direct melatonin-glomerular interaction should not be ignored. Indeed, in recent immunoblotting experiments, we have been able to demonstrate the presence of MR in primary cultures of human mesangial cells (Song and Silverman, unpublished results).

Given the complexity of melatonin interactions with different cells in the kidney through its specific receptors, the superimposed modulatory activity of other cross-reacting hormones, and the great species variability, it will take a lot more work before a clear picture emerges of how melatonin influences renal function.

Acknowledgments

Y. Song is supported by a fellowship from the Kidney Foundation of Canada. The research was supported by an MRC Membrane Biology Group grant to M. Silverman

References

1. Zrenner, C., Theories of pineal function from classical antiquity to 1900: a history, in Reiter, R.J.R., Ed., *Pineal Research Review,* Vol. 3, Alan R. Liss, New York, 1985, 1.

2. Binkley, S., Introduction, in Binkley, S., Ed., *The Pineal: Endocrine and Nonendocrine Function,* Prentice Hall, Englewood Cliffs, NJ, 1988, 1.

3. Lerner, A.B., Case, J.D., Takahashi, Y., Lee, T.H., and Mori, W., Isolation of mela-tonin, the pineal gland factor that lightens melanocytes, *J. Am. Chem. Soc.* 80, 2587, 1958.

4. Lerner, A.B., Case, J.D., and Heinzelman, R.V., Structure of melatonin, *J. Am. Chem. Soc.,* 81, 6084, 1959.

5. Quay, W.B., Circadian rhythm in rat pineal serotonin and its modification by estrous scycle and photoperiod, *Gen. Comp. Endocrinol.,* 3, 473, 1963.

6. Wurtman, R.J., Axelrod, J., and Phillips, L.S., Melatonin synthesis in the pineal gland: control by light, *Science,* 142, 1071, 1963.

7. Wurtman, R.J., Axelrod, H., and Fischer, J.E., Melatonin synthesis in the pineal gland: effect of light mediated by the sympathetic nervous system, *Science,* 143, 1328, 1964.

8. Reiter, R.J.R. and Hester, R.J., Interrelationships of the pineal gland, the superior cervical ganglia and the photoperiod in the regulation of the endocrine systems of hamsters, *Endocrinology,* 79, 1168, 1965.

9. Brown, G.M., Chronopharmacological actions of the pineal gland, *Drug Metab. Drug Interact.,* 8, 189, 1990

10. Pang, S.F., Lee, P.P.N., Chan, Y.S., and Ayre, E.A., Melatonin secretion and its rhythms in biological fluids, in Yu, H.S. and Reiter, R.J.R., Eds., *Melatonin: Biosynthesis, Physiological Effects and Clinical Applications*, CRC Press, Boca Raton, FL, 1993, 129.

11. Reiter, R.J.R., The melatonin rhythm: both a clock and a calendar, *Experientia,* 49, 654, 1993.

12. Reiter, R.J.R., The pineal and its hormones in the control of reproduction in mammals, *Endocrine Rev.*, 1, 109, 1980.

13. Brown, G.M., Tsui, H.W., Niles, L.P., and Grota, L.J., Gonadal effects of the pineal gland, in Kennaway, C.K. and Seamark, R.F., Eds., *The Pineal Gland*, Elsevier/North Holland Biomedical Press, New York, 1982, 89.

14. Reiter, R.J.R., Pineal melatonin: cell biology of its synthesis and its physiological interactions, *Endocrine Rev.*, 12, 151, 1991.

15. Rosolowska-Huszca, D., Thaela, M.J., Jagura, M., Stepien, D., and Skwarlo-Sonta, K., Pineal influence on the diurnal rhythm of nonspecific immunity indoles in chickens, *J. Pineal Res.* 10, 190, 1991.

16. Skwarlo-Sonta, K., Thaela, M. J., Midura, M., Lech, B., Gluchowska, B., Drela, N., Kozlowska, E., and Kowalczyk, R., Exogenous melatonin modifies the circadian rhythm but does not increase the level of some immune parameters in the chicken, *J. Pineal Res.*, 12, 27, 1992.

17. Maestroni, G.J.M., The immunoneuroendocrine role of melatonin, *J. Pineal Res.*, 14, 1, 1993.

18. Karppanen, H., and Vapaatalo, H., Effects of aldosterone antagonist, spironolactone, on pinealectomized rats, *Pharmacology,* 6, 257, 1971.

19. Richardson, B.A., Studier, E.H., Stallone, J.N., and Kennedy, C.M., Effects of melatonin on water metabolism and renal function in male Syrian hamsters (*Mesocricetus auratus*), *J. Pineal Res.*, 13, 49, 1992.

20. Pang, C.S., Tang, P.L., Song, Y., Brown, G.M., and Pang, S.F., 2-[125I]Iiodomelatonin binding sites in the quail heart: characteristics, distribution and modulation by guanine nucleotides and cations, *Life Sci.,* 58, 1047, 1996.

21. Viswanathan, M., Hissa, R., and George, J.C., Effects of short photoperiod and melatonin treatment on thermogenesis in the Syrian hamster, *J. Pineal Res.*, 3, 311, 1986.

22. John, T.M., Itoh, S., and George, J.C., On the role of the pineal in thermoregulation in the pigeon, *Horm. Res.*, 9, 41, 1978.

23. Ralph, C.L., Firth, B.T., Gern, W.K., and Owens, D.W., The pineal complex and thermoregulation, *Biol. Rev.*, 54, 41, 1979.

24. Song, Y., Chan, C.W.Y., Brown, G.M., Pang, S.F., and Silverman, M., Studies of the renal action of melatonin: evidence that the effects are mediated by 37-kDa receptors of the Mel-1a subtype localized primarily to the basolateral membrane of the proximal tubule, *FASEB J.,* 11, 93, 1997.

25. Ng, T.B., Effect of pineal indoles on corticosterone and aldosterone production by isolated rat adrenal cells, *Biochem. Int.*, 14, 635, 1987.

26. Niles, L.P., Brown, G.M., and Grota L.J., Endocrine effects of the pineal gland and neutralization of circulating melatonin and *N*-acetylserotonin, *Can. J. Physiol. Pharmacol.*, 55, 537, 1977.

27. Rebuffat, P., Kanchev, L.N., and Stankov, B.M., Effect of melatonin on steroid production by rat adrenals under *in vitro* superfusion conditions, *Life Sci.*, 44, 1955, 1989.

28. Vaughan, G.M., Vaughan, M.K., and Mason, A.D., Comparison of thyroid hormones and testes weight across pineal-related perturbations, in Brown, G.M. and Wainwright, S.D., Eds., *The Pineal Gland: Endocrine Aspects*, Pergamon Press, Oxford, 1985, 257.

29. Demine, C. and Kritzler, J.S., Pineal involvement in the effects of short photoperiods on thyroid follicular cells in the Syrian hamster, in Brown, G.M. and Wainwright, S.D. Eds., *The Pineal Gland: Endocrine Aspects*, Pergamon Press, Oxford, 1985, 265.

30. Bubenik, G.A. and Pang, S.F., The role of serotonin and melatonin in gastrointestinal physiology: ontogeny, regulation of food intake, and mutual serotonin-melatonin feedback, *J. Pineal Res.* 16, 91, 1994.

31. Chow, P.H., Lee, P.N., Poon, A.M.S., Shiu, S.Y.W., and Pang S.F., The gastrointestinal system: a site of melatonin paracrine action, in *Frontiers in Hormone Research*, Vol. 21, *Melatonin: A Universal Photoperiodic Signal with Diverse Actions*, Tang, P.L., Pang, S.F., and Reiter, R.J.R., Eds., Karger, Basel, 1996, 123.

32. Vakkuri, O., Lamsa, E., Rahkamaa, E., Ruotsalainen, H., and Leppaluoto, J., Iodinated melatonin: preparation and characterization of the molecular structure by mass or 1H NMR spectroscopy, *Analyt. Biochem.*, 142, 284, 1984.

33. Vanecek, J., Pavlik, A., and Illnerova, H., Hypothalamic melatonin receptor sites revealed by autoradiography, *Brain Res.*, 435, 359, 1987.

34. Dubocovich, M.L., Pharmacology and function of melatonin receptors, *FASEB J.*, 2, 2765, 1988.

35. Pang, S.F., Dubocovich, M.L., and Brown, G.M., Melatonin receptors in peripheral tissues: a new area of melatonin research, *Biol. Signals*, 54, 177, 1993.

36. Ebisawa, T., Karne, S., Lerner, M.R., and Reppert, S.M., Expression cloning of a high-affinity melatonin receptor from *Xenopus* dermal melanophores, *Proc. Natl. Acad. Sci. USA*, 91, 6133, 1994.

37. Reppert, S.M., Weaver, D.R., and Ebisawa, T., Cloning and characterization of a mammalian melatonin receptor that mediates reproductive and circadian responses, *Neuron*, 13, 1177, 1994.

38. Reppert, S.M., Godson, D., Mahle, C.D., Weaver, D.R., Slaugenhaupt, S.A., and Gusella, J.F., Molecular characterization of a second melatonin receptor expressed in human retina and brain: the Mel-1b melatonin receptor, *Proc. Natl. Acad. Sci. USA*, 92, 8734, 1995.

39. Reppert, S.M., Weaver, D.R., Cassone, V.M., Godson, C., and Kolakowski, Jr., L.F., Melatonin receptors are for the birds: molecular analysis of two receptor subtypes deferentially expressed in chick brain, *Neuron*, 15, 1003, 1995.

40. Liu, F., Yuan, H., Sugamori, K.S., Hamadanizadeh, A., Lee, F.J.S., Pang, S.F., Brown, G.M., Pristupa, Z.B., and Niznik, H.B., Molecular and functional characterization of a partial cDNA encoding a novel chicken brain melatonin receptor, *FEBS Lett.*, 347, 273, 1995.

41. Dubocovich, M.L., Melatonin receptors: are there multiple subtypes?, *Trends Pharmacol. Sci.*, 16, 50, 1995.

42. Barbarossa, C., Demartino, C., Peruzy, D., and Torlonia, G., The pituitary-pineal antagonism, *Acta Endocr.,* Suppl. 51, 79, 1960.

43. Arutyunyan, G.S., Mashkovskii, M.D., and Roshchina, L.F., Pharmacological properties of melatonin, *Farmakologiya i. Toksikologiya,* 26, T1330, 1963.

44. Machado, A.B.M. and Da Silva, C.R., Pineal body and urinary sodium excretion in the rat, *Experientia,* 19, 264, 1963.

45. Csaba, G. and Bûkay, J., The effect of melatonin and corpus pineal extract on serum electrolytes in the rat, *Acta Biol. Acad. Sci. Hung.,* 28, 143, 1977.

46. Tsuda, T., Ide, M., and Ligo, M., Influences of season and of temperature, photoperiod and subcutaneous melatonin infusion on the glomerular filtration rate of ewes, *J. Pineal Res.,* 19, 166, 1995.

47. Morton, D.J., Effect of methoxyindole administration on plasma cation levels in the rat, *J. Pineal Res.,* 6, 141, 1989.

48. Morton, D.J., Alteration of plasma cation levels in rats kept in constant light, *J. Pineal Res.,* 9, 95, 1990.

49. Koopman, M.G., Minors, D.S., and Waterhouse, J.M., Urinary and renal circadian rhythms, in Adrendt, J., Minors, D.S., and Waterhouse, J.M., Eds., *Biological Rhythms in Clinical Practice,* Wright, London, 1989, 83.

50. Koopman, M.G., Koomen, G.C., van Aeker, B.A., and Arisz, L., Urinary sodium excretion in patients with nephrotic syndrome and its circadian variation, *Q. J. Med.,* 87, 109, 1994.

51. Kemp, G.J., Blumsohn, A., and Morris, B.W., Circadian changes in plasma phosphate concentration, urinary phosphate excretion and cellular phosphate shifts, *Clin. Chem.,* 38, 400, 1992.

52. Song, Y., Ayre, E.A., and Pang, S.F., The identification and characterization of ^{125}I-labelled iodomelatonin-binding sites in the duck kidney, *J. Endocrinol.,* 135, 353, 1992.

53. Song, Y., Poon, A.M.S., Lee, P.P.N., and Pang, S.F., Putative melatonin receptors in the male guinea pig kidney, *J. Pineal Res.,* 15, 153, 1993.

54. Song, Y., Tam, P.C., Poon, A.M.S., Brown, G.M., and Pang, S.F., 2-[125I]Iodomelatonin binding sites in the human kidney and the effect of guanosine 5′-O-(3-thiotriphosphate), *J. Clin. Endocrinol. Metab.,* 80, 1560, 1995.

55. Song, Y., Pang, C.S., Ayre, E.A., Brown, G.M., and Pang, S.F., Melatonin receptors in the chicken kidney: up-regulated by pinealectomy and integrated with adenylate cyclase, *Eur. J. Endocrinol.,* 135, 128, 1996.

56. Song, Y., Ayre, E.A., and Pang, S.F., [125I]Iodomelatonin binding sites in mammalian and avian kidneys (review), *Biol. Signals,* 2, 207, 1993.

57. Drew, J.E., Williams, L.M., Hannah, L.T., Barrett, P., Abramovich, D.R., and Morgan, P.J., Localization and characterization of melatonin receptors in the human fetal kidney, *J. Endocrinol.,* 151, 76, 1996.

58. Song, Y., Poon, A.M.S., Brown, G.M., and Pang, S.F., Ontogeny of 2-[125I]iodomelatonin binding sites in the kidney and spleen of chicken (*Gallus domesticus*), *Can. J. Pharm. Physiol.,* 73, 685, 1995.

59. Brown, G.M., Pang, S.F., Silverman, M., Chan, C.W.Y., and Song, Y., Melatonin receptors in kidney and other peripheral tissues, in Webbs, S., Puig-Domingo, M., Muller, M., and Pevet, P., Eds., *Pineal Gland Update 1996: From Molecular Biology to Clinical Medicine*, PJD Publications, New York, pp. 203–211.

60. Chan, C.W.Y., Song, Y., Ailenberg, M., Wheeler, M., Pang, S.F., Brown, G.M., and Silverman, M., Studies of melatonin effects on epithelia using the human embryonic kidney-293 (HEK-293) cell line, *Endocrinology*, 188, 4732, 1997.

61. Song, Y., Lee, P.J.P.N., Chan, C.W.Y., Brown, G.M., Pang, S.F., and Silverman, M., Current advances in renal melatonin receptors, in Tang, P.L., Pang, S.F., and Reiter, R.J.R., Eds., *Frontiers in Hormone Research*, Vol. 21, *Melatonin: A Universal Photoperiodic Signal with Diverse Actions*, Karger, Basel, 1996, 115.

62. Conway, S., Drew, J.E., Canning, S.J., Barrett, P., Jockers, R., Strosberg, A.D., Guardiola-Lemaitre, B., Delagrange, P., and Morgan, P.J., Identification of Mel-1a melatonin receptors in the human embryonic kidney cell line HEK293: evidence of G protein-coupled melatonin receptors which do not mediate the inhibition of stimulated cyclic AMP levels, *FEBS Lett.*, 407, 121, 1997.

Chapter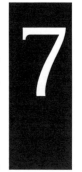

Melatonin and Seasonal Changes in Body Fat

Timothy J. Bartness and Jacqueline B. Fine

Contents

Introduction

Environmental influences are recognized as important factors contributing to the etiology of human obesity.[1] Although this point might seem obvious, the role of the environment in energy regulation is under-represented in nonhuman animal models of human energy balance disorders. For example, the predominant animal models for obesity research are based on genetic, not environmental, factors.[2] Considerable knowledge about the development and maintenance of the obese state has been gleaned using these genetic models; however, knowledge about body fat loss has not been forthcoming from these models because genetic obesity is nonreversible. We and others have suggested that animals showing annual food intake and body mass (fat) cycles also may be valuable for understanding human obesity and eating disorders because these obesities are naturally reversible.[3–5] Why do some animals show seasonal responses in energy balance and other changes such as the ability to reproduce?

It often is critical for animals that live in temperate zones to prepare for future changes in the season so that biologically important physiological and behavioral responses occur at an optimal time of year. For example, significant decreases in the ambient temperature and forageable food associated with winter make the rearing of offspring even more energetically challenging than normal for these species.[6] Two general categories emerge among species showing seasonal responses: (1) species that respond primarily to changes in the photoperiod (day length), such as hamsters and voles, and (2) species that respond to the timing of an endogenous "clock" of unknown location, such as ground squirrels, woodchucks, and marmots.[7–9] Species in the latter category have body and lipid mass, and reproductive cycles of approximately 1 year (i.e., circannual rhythms). In contrast, in the former species, most of the seasonally adaptive responses, such as alterations in reproductive status, pelage (coat) color, and energy balance (energy expenditure vs. energy intake), are triggered by changes in the day length.[4,10,11] Photoperiod-induced changes in white adipose tissue (WAT), the major energy storage depot for mammals,[12] and brown adipose tissue (BAT), a major site of heat generation (energy expenditure) in mammals,[13] have been studied in a relatively small number of species. The most extensively investigated species for both adipose tissues include Syrian and Siberian hamsters (for a review, see Reference 4) and several species of voles and lemmings. Therefore, this review will highlight these hamster species because they are used in the preponderance of these studies. The seasonally adaptive changes in these adipose tissues and in the gonads take weeks or months to be manifested fully or to become functional. Therefore, it appears that natural selection has favored animals that can accurately begin these responses before the heart of the next season. How do animals "know" what season is forthcoming?

The most noise-free signal of the transition between seasons is the change in the photoperiod (day length).[14] Indeed, these seasonally adaptive responses can be triggered in the laboratory, regardless of the time of year, simply by changing the duration of light exposure.[15,16] For example, hamster and vole species will show the full complement of short day (SD) photoperiod ("winter-like") responses if the day length is significantly shortened.[17] How is the photoperiod cue transduced into a biological signal within the organism?

The photoperiod cue is received by the retina and transmitted through a multisynaptic pathway to the pineal gland beginning with the retinal ganglion cells in mammals.[18] Interruption of this circuit at any point, including the eyes and the pineal, will result in a blockade of the effects of SDs on the reproductive system[18] and most other seasonal responses, including changes in the level of adiposity.[4,19] For example, pinealectomy blocks the photoperiod-dependent changes in body and lipid mass in Syrian hamsters,[19] although evidence for a photoperiod-induced, pineal-*independent* effect also has been reported.[19,20] Pinealectomy also blocks the seasonal changes in body and lipid mass of Siberian hamsters[21–23] and meadow voles.[24,25] Once the neurochemical rendition of the photic stimulus reaches the pinealocytes, it is transduced into an endocrine signal in the form of the rhythmic pattern of secretion of the hormone, melatonin (MEL). Pineal and plasma melatonin concentrations are at their daily nadir during the light phase of the photocycle and at their peak during portions of the dark phase.[10,26] This pattern of melatonin synthesis and secretion results from the regulation of the pineal gland by an endogenous circadian oscillator that is entrained to the light/dark cycle.[27] Thus, the duration of the night is coded by the duration of the secretion of MEL and serves to trigger seasonal responses — long-duration MEL secretion profiles signal "fall/winter", whereas short-duration MEL secretion profiles signal "spring/summer".[10]

Initially, the critical nature of the duration of the MEL signal for triggering changes in reproductive status was demonstrated by giving LD-housed, pineal-intact Syrian hamsters daily s.c. injections of MEL 2 to 3 hr before lights-out (i.e., the so-called "timed afternoon injection paradigm").[28] The rationale underlying the use of this paradigm is that the afternoon injections of exogenous MEL cause circulating MEL concentrations to rise and summate with the endogenous nocturnal peak of the hormone. This results in an overall lengthening of the MEL signal beyond its naturally occurring LD length and, consequently, the elicitation of SD-like gonadal regression.[28] The importance of the peak duration of the MEL secretion profile for triggering SD responses was demonstrated more conclusively using juvenile and adult Siberian hamsters, adult Syrian hamsters, and sheep and employing the "timed infusion" paradigm (TIP).[10] In this paradigm, the animals are pinealectomized (to remove the endogenous secretion of MEL) and then infused with MEL peripherally to permit manipulations of the various components of the MEL secretion profile, such as duration, amplitude, and the time of day of the signal. The resulting serum concentrations of MEL can be made to occur within the physiological range for this hormone,[29] unlike the supraphysiological concentrations of the hormone that result from the doses of MEL required to elicit SD-like responses using the timed afternoon injection paradigm.[30] Most importantly for the theme of this review, the TIP has been used to show a similar critical nature of the peak duration of the MEL secretion profile for the photoperiod-induced changes in body and lipid mass.[22,23,31,32] Where is the MEL signal received, and how does it affect photoperiod-sensitive peripheral tissues?

There are populations of MEL receptors suggested by the binding of a radioactive MEL analog (2-[^{125}I]iodomelatonin; IMEL) to brain tissue.[33–35] IMEL central nervous system (CNS) binding sites have been reported in a wide range of mammals (i.e., sheep; deer; goats; rabbits; laboratory rats; Syrian, Siberian, and European hamsters; white-footed mice; golden-mantled ground squirrels; guinea pigs; nine-banded armadillos; humans), as well as in other animals (Atlantic hagfish, lamprey, hedgehog skates, rainbow trout, clawed toads).[33] In mammals, one brain site and one peripherally located site consistently show IMEL binding — the suprachiasmatic nucleus of the hypothalamus (SCN) and the pars tuberalis (PT) of the pituitary gland, respectively.[36–39] Many of the mammals examined to date show binding in both SCN and the PT; however, some seasonally breeding species show only IMEL binding in the PT.[40,41] The presence of mRNA for the physiologically active MEL receptor, the Mel-1a receptor, has been observed in the SCN and PT of Siberian hamsters and laboratory rats.[42] Which of these receptor populations receives the MEL signal and participates in the photoperiod-induced changes in body and lipid mass?

Although the answer to this question is far from known at this time, it appears that the SCN is at least one site important for the MEL-induced changes in reproductive status, and body and lipid mass. Thus, pinealectomized Siberian,[43] but not Syrian,[44] hamsters bearing SCN lesions receiving daily SD-like MEL signals via the TIP exhibit SD-induced gonadal regression and decreased body and WAT pad masses. What is not known is to which other brain structures the information contained within the MEL signals is transmitted. It is known, however, that the rostral projections of the nuclei to the PVN and sub-PVN areas,[32] or the dorsomedial/dorsocaudal SCN projections to the PVT and other brain sites,[31] are not necessary for the transmission of the information contained in the MEL signals. These conclusions were reached based on microknife cuts that severed these SCN efferent projections in pinealectomized Siberian hamsters that received SD MEL signals via the TIP. Further studies are needed to define which neurons within the SCN receive MEL signals and how these signals are transmitted and processed such that changes in reproductive and adipose tissues result. To this end, preliminary data indicate that Mel-1a receptor mRNA is co-localized with arginine vasopressin (AVP) in the SCN of Siberian hamsters (Song, Bartness, and Bittman, unpublished observations). Because MEL does not seem to have direct effects on the gonads or adipose tissue,[45] ultimately MEL signals must be transduced into hormonal or neural signals that affect these, and other, peripheral tissues. How are the potential hormonal intermediaries for the effects of MEL on peripheral tissues, especially WAT and BAT, identified?

First, photoperiod-induced changes in hormone concentration are determined experimentally, then a classic experimental strategy typically is used to test the roles of these hormones. Specifically, in terms of the latter, serum concentrations of the hormones are created that are opposite to those that prevail normally in the photoperiod. The results of the experiments described below include the description of the photoperiod-induced changes in each hormone, if it is known, and the use of this and other experimental tactics. These approaches have been most extensively examined in Siberian hamsters and to a lesser degree Syrian hamsters and voles. Therefore, these species will be the primary focus of this review, although other species such as deer mice, European hamsters, and lemmings also will be included where appropriate.

Gonadal Steroids

It is important to note that, although hamsters,[46–49] voles,[50,51] collared lemmings,[52] and deer mice[53,54] regress their gonads in response to SD exposure, their body and lipid mass responses differ (see below). That is, collared lemmings,[55] prairie voles,[56] and Syrian hamsters[19,57,58] *increase* their body and lipid mass when exposed to SDs, whereas Siberian hamsters,[48,49,59–61] European hamsters,[47] meadow voles,[51,62] and deer mice[63,64] all exhibit SD-induced *decreases* in their body and lipid masses. The degree of these SD-induced changes in body mass and fat varies among these species and, within each species, also varies between the sexes (see below). The SD-triggered alterations in body and lipid mass can often be predicted by the effects of gonadectomy in LD-housed individuals in some of these species, perhaps because both conditions result in decreased testosterone (T) in males and estrogen (E_2) in females. For example, LD-housed female Syrian hamsters,[65,66] female collared lemmings,[55] and male prairie voles[56] increase their body and lipid masses when they are gonadectomized and consequently show similar responses when "photoperiodically gonadectomized".[19,55,56] In contrast, Siberian hamsters,[61,67] male deer mice,[68] meadow voles,[62,69] and European hamsters[47,70] decrease their body and lipid masses when gonadectomized, an effect mimicked by SD exposure.[47–49,51,59–62,64,70,71] On an individual basis, these generalized body and lipid mass responses after gonadectomy may require qualification, at least for one of these species; when LD-housed male meadow voles with the heaviest body masses are castrated, they decrease their body masses, whereas when LD-housed male meadow voles with the lightest body masses are castrated, they increase their body masses.[69] In these cases, replacement of T also produces the opposite effects of gonadectomy. That is, the formerly heavy voles that lost body mass with castration increase body mass with T treatment and vice versa for formerly light voles.[69] For the other species that lose body and lipid mass with SD exposure (i.e., Siberian hamsters, deer mice), treatment with gonadal steroids reverses or blocks the effects of gonadectomy.[21,64,67,72,73]

The simplest interpretation of the general effects of SD exposure on body and lipid mass is that the increases or decreases in these responses are secondary to the primary effect of the SD-induced regression of their gonads, an effect that is complete after approximately 5 to 8 weeks of SD exposure. The photoperiod/MEL-induced changes in body and lipid mass are not, however, merely due to a "photoperiod-produced gonadectomy" because a large percentage of the SD-induced changes in body and lipid mass are independent of regression of the gonads (see below for details). In addition, for those species that have been studied, the spontaneous recrudescence of their body and/or lipid masses (i.e., a return to LD status despite continued, long-term SD exposure [usually >20 wk]) also is partly independent of the gonadal responses. That is, in addition to the spontaneous recrudescence of the gonads, body and lipid masses return to their LD levels in both gonad-intact and gonadectomized animals. Specifically, ovariectomized Syrian hamsters,[74] castrated male European hamsters,[47] castrated male meadow voles,[62] and cold-exposed castrated male Siberian hamsters[73] all show reversal of their species-specific increases or decreases in their body and/ or lipid mass responses to SDs despite being gonadectomized. In addition, if SD-housed, castrated, male Siberian hamsters at their body mass nadir are abruptly shifted to LDs, they show a nearly identical increase in body mass compared to SD-housed testes-intact hamsters experiencing identical changes in the photoperiod.[75]

The mechanisms that underlie the SD MEL-induced body and lipid mass responses that are secondary to the "physiological gonadectomy" are not well understood. Our understanding is improving concerning how the photoperiod/MEL changes in WAT and brown adipose tissue seem to support the preparation of some animals, especially Syrian hamsters, for overwintering. Specifically, SD exposure of male Syrian hamsters markedly decreases (−84%) the number of adrenergic receptors on their WAT adipocyte (fat cell) membranes that oppose decreases in body fat by countering the mobilization (lipolysis) of lipid stores from these cells.[76] This SD-induced decrease in "antilipolytic" receptors, the α_2-adrenergic receptors, parallels the SD-induced decreases in serum T.[76] Moreover, the SD-triggered decreases in WAT α_2-adrenergic receptors are reversed by T replacement treatment.[76] These changes in adrenergic receptor only affect the α_2-adrenergic receptors and not any of the β-adrenergic receptors nor the α_1 receptors[78] and are due to a direct action of T (not to aromatization of T) on these receptors.[79] Furthermore, castrated male Syrian hamsters show castration-induced decreases in the activity of the WAT enzyme responsible for uptake of fatty acids into adipocytes, lipoprotein lipase.[66] Together, these changes in WAT appear to support a condition conducive for the mobilization of lipid fuels, rather than their storage, by WAT. This condition could supply fat-derived fuels to cope with declining ambient temperatures and decreases in forageable food sources. In addition, the SD-induced increase in BAT thermogenic capacity (increase in mitochondrial cytochrome-C-oxidase activity), thermogenic status (GDP-binding) and decrease in activity of the sympathetic nervous system (SNS) drive on BAT (norepinephrine turnover) might represent conditions of BAT that would adapt it for the forthcoming thermogenic challenges faced by overwintering animals. Central nervous system sites that are the brain origins of the SNS innervation of BAT and WAT[80,81] and that might be instrumental in these and other sympathetically mediated changes in lipid metabolism specifically, and energy balance generally, are discussed briefly below and in more detail elsewhere.[82]

Prolactin

The general role of prolactin (PRL) in lipid metabolism is not well understood, but at least in some small mammalian species, such as laboratory rats, PRL appears capable of altering lipid fuel stores in WAT *in vivo* and *in vitro*.[83,84] All species exhibiting photoperiod/MEL control of reproductive cycles, regardless of whether they are LD or SD breeders,[85,86] show SD-induced decreased PRL secretion/serum concentrations. An important role for the photoperiodic/MEL regulation of lipid deposition or mobilization by PRL, however, has not been clearly demonstrated. For example, Syrian and Siberian hamsters show the typical SD-induced decreases in serum PRL concentrations;[86–88] however, elevation of serum PRL concentrations in SD-housed Syrian and Siberian hamsters through implantation of LD pituitaries, or by infusion of ovine PRL, respectively, does not result in decreases or increases in lipid mass or changes in WAT metabolism.[89] Moreover, injections of the dopamine receptor agonist (and therefore PRL secretion inhibitor) bromocryptine (CB-154) to LD-housed Syrian and Siberian hamsters does not result in species-specific SD-like changes in lipid mass or WAT metabolism.[89] Similarly, infusions of ovine PRL, designed to produce LD serum concentrations of the PRL, do not increase body and fat pad masses to LD levels.[89,90] This treatment does, however, trigger the growth of a summer-like pelage,[89–92] demonstrating the bioactivity of the non-native PRL (ovine) in this species. Therefore, at least in Syrian and Siberian hamsters, it does not appear that PRL is a significant mediator of photoperiod/MEL-induced changes in body and lipid mass. It should be noted, however, that a critical role for PRL in the development of photoperiod-induced, seasonal changes in body fat[93–97] has been reported by one laboratory, but not supported by the findings of others.[90,98] Finally, experimental hyperprolactinemia, produced by multiple pituitary explants, can block the SD-induced changes in BAT in Syrian hamsters.[99]

Thyroid Hormones

The pineal gland and MEL clearly modulate the neuroendocrine-thyroid gland axis and, consequently, the secretion of thyroxine (T_4) and triiodothyronine (T_3) in a variety of species.[100] In LD-breeding small rodents, SD exposure decreases serum concentrations of T_4 and T_3 in Syrian hamsters[101,102] and collared lemmings.[103,104] More modest SD-induced decreases in these hormones are seen in Siberian hamsters.[105–107] Collectively, these SD-induced reductions in thyroid hormones are somewhat surprising because winter-like SDs would typically be associated with decreases in ambient temperature in the wild. Because most rodent species increase their secretion of thyroid hormones in response to cold exposure,[108] it may be that the neuroendocrine-thyroid axis is stimulated in these animals only when they are actually cold-exposed, but not in preparation for cold exposure. A clear role for thyroid hormones in the photoperiod-induced changes in body fat has not been shown experimentally, despite the regulation of the thyroid gland by the photoperiod/MEL.[104] Specifically, SD-housed male Siberian hamsters given daily T_4 injections have LD-like serum T_4 and T_3 concentrations, yet show decreases in body, fat pad, and paired testes masses that are similar to those of SD-housed vehicle- and non-injected hamsters.[107] Therefore, photoperiod/MEL-induced changes in thyroid hormones do not seem to have a major role in the seasonal control of body and lipid mass, especially in these hamster species.

Glucocorticoids

The role of the glucocorticoids in the photoperiod/MEL-controlled alterations in energy balance has been infrequently addressed. The role of glucocorticoids in the regulation of energy balance (including food intake, lipid mobilization, and storage) and thermogenesis is well established in four typically studied models of human obesity (diet, genetic, endocrine, and hypothalamic).[109] Glucocorticoid secretion after changes in the photoperiod has been shown for some of the rodent species discussed above. For example, Syrian[102,110] and Siberian[111] hamsters, prairie voles,[112] and collared lemmings[104] show seasonal changes in serum cortisol or corticosterone concentrations, or changes in both (note that unlike laboratory rats[113,114] or humans,[115] hamsters have significant serum concentrations of both hormones).[102,110,111,116] To our knowledge, experimental manipulation of type II glucocorticoid receptors found on adipocytes[117] only has been performed in one species showing photoperiod/MEL-induced changes in adiposity — Siberian hamsters. The type II glucocorticoid receptor blocker RU486[111] was used because it does not act as a progestin receptor blocker in hamsters[118] and because adrenalectomy cannot be used to manipulate glucocorticoids in hamsters — hamsters do not show a salt appetite when adrenalectomized and consequently do not thrive and frequently die after surgery. RU486 was administered via constant-release implants to LD-housed male Siberian hamsters in an attempt to produce a SD-like glucocorticoid environment. Trends towards SD-like decreases in inguinal WAT (IWAT) and epididymal WAT (EWAT) mass were seen in RU486-treated hamsters. Body mass and carcass lipid content were significantly decreased at the highest dose of RU486, although the decrease in carcass lipid content was accompanied by a similar decrease in carcass water content, the latter not normally associated with photoperiod/MEL-induced decreases in body mass in this species.[61,67,119] Therefore, unlike the effects of blockade of type II glucocorticoid receptors by RU486 in genetic- and diet-induced obesity in laboratory rats,[120,121] these receptors, and perhaps glucocorticoids in general, do not seem to be a primary factor in the photoperiodic/MEL control of seasonal body and lipid mass cycles, at least in the one species studied. It would seem interesting to test whether RU486 would block the SD-induced increase in body and lipid mass in female Syrian hamsters.

Insulin, Growth Hormone, Somatomedins, and Glucagon

Relative to the study of gonadal steroid and thyroid hormones, or PRL discussed above, the roles of insulin, growth hormone, somatomedins, and glucagon have been examined infrequently in the attempts to determine the hormonal intermediary for the effects of photoperiod/MEL on body and lipid masses. Below, we will review the few data that have been presented on this topic.

To our knowledge, of the species discussed above that show photoperiodic control of reproductive cycles, the effects of SD exposure on serum insulin concentrations have only been documented in Syrian and Siberian hamsters. Specifically, SD exposure causes decreases in serum insulin concentrations in Siberian hamsters[116] and increases in serum insulin concentration in Syrian hamsters.[94–96,122] In Siberian hamsters, serum insulin concentrations are decreased fourfold in SD-housed hamsters compared with their LD-housed counterparts.[116] These findings seem congruent with the well-studied relation between serum insulin concentrations and the level of adiposity.[123,124] Serum insulin concentrations clamped from the physiological to supraphysiological levels have been created experimentally in Siberian hamsters. Specifically, low, near physiological serum concentrations of the hormone were created by inducing experimental diabetes mellitus via injections of the beta cell toxin streptozotocin and giving varying levels of insulin replacement,[125] whereas high supraphysiological serum concentrations of the hormone were created by giving insulin in several doses to non-diabetic control hamsters.[116] These treatments produced a wide range of LD body masses that were positively correlated with insulin status. All groups exhibited normal gonadal regression, decreases in body and lipid mass, and food intake when transferred to SDs. Although the LD baseline body masses were quite disparate for animals at these extremes of serum insulin concentrations, all groups reached the same body and lipid mass nadir after exposure to SDs.[116,125] Collectively, these data suggest that insulin status does not play a major role in the photoperiodic control of adiposity that body and/or lipid mass is "protected" at a minimum level after SD exposure for this species.

The only study to examine the role of insulin in the SD-induced increase in the level of fatness in Syrian hamsters used total subdiaphragmatic vagotomy to block the neural control of insulin secretion by the parasympathetic nervous system and to eliminate sensory efferent information from peripheral organs (e.g., stomach, intestines, liver) to the brain.[122] Vagotomized hamsters did not show SD-induced increases in body and lipid mass and food intake, although they did exhibit gonadal regression.[122] Interpretation of these data relative to the role of insulin in the SD-induced increases in body and lipid mass in this species is difficult because total subdiapharagmatic vagotomy causes a multitude of effects,[126] not just blockade of the neural control of the pancreas.

The role of growth hormone (GH) and insulin-like growth factors (somatomedins) in the photoperiodic control of body and lipid mass has not received much attention in the investigation of potential hormonal intermediaries of MEL. Collared lemmings show increases in body mass in SDs associated with increases in GH.[103,104] Syrian hamsters do not show changes in serum GH concentrations when transferred from LDs to SDs,[127,128] but timed afternoon MEL injections increase GH secretion,[129] increase body and lipid mass,[19,74] and regress the gonads in this species.[28] This effect of MEL injections on serum GH concentrations seems puzzling given the lack of effect of SDs on this hormone.

Insulin-like growth factor-1 (IGF-1) is found in the circulation and in many tissues, including WAT.[130–132] IGF-1 has a pronounced effect on WAT pre-adipocyte (i.e., stromal-vascular cells) differentiation[132,133] and, in this manner, could affect photoperiod-induced chantes in adipocyte cellularity. Although it has been argued that the reversibility of SD-induced obesity in Syrian hamsters occurs because there are no increases in fat cell number (FCN),[74,134] we have seen increases in FCN in the parametrial WAT, IWAT, and EWAT pads of SD-exposed female Syrian hamsters, in addition to increases in fat cell size (volume) also were seen in all pads. The possible role of IGF-1 in the SD-induced increase in WAT FCN is supported by the finding that timed afternoon injections of MEL in Syrian hamsters produce twofold increases in serum IGF-1 concentrations.[129,135]

The pancreatic and intestinal hormone glucagon is well known for its lipolytic effects on WAT and stimulation of BAT thermogenesis. To our knowledge, serum levels of glucagon have not been measured in any of the species that show seasonal reproductive cycles controlled by the photoperiod discussed above; however, it seems likely that glucagon may play a significant role in the photoperiodic control of energy balance. For example, glucagon stimulates BAT thermogenesis[136] and is an important hormone in the thermogenic response to the cold.[137] In addition, WAT has glucagon receptors,[138] thus providing an additional means by which lipolysis can be controlled independent of its control by the sympathetic nervous system (see below). Therefore, it may be that SD-induced increases in glucagon secretion in species that exhibit SD-induced decreases in body and lipid mass, such as Siberian hamsters, could account for some of the mobilization of lipid stores from WAT as well as increases in the thermogenic capacity of BAT in these animals.[136,139]

Summary of the Search for the Hormonal Intermediary for Melatonin

Although the studies have not been exhaustive, the effects of any single hormone do not seem to account for the photoperiod-induced changes in body and lipid mass responses. It is possible, of course, that changes in a constellation of hormones are necessary to produce these and other photoperiodic responses. Such studies are not only demanding in terms of the possible combinations of hormones to test, but also are technically difficult in that many of the hormones affected by the photoperiod/ MEL exhibit 24-hr variations in their secretion and metabolism. Thus, the ability to mimic accurately the natural secretion profile for pairs, triplets, or quartets of these hormones is difficult or impossible. Alternatively, it may be that MEL signals affect WAT and BAT through innervation originating in the CNS. What is the evidence for the innervation of these adipose tissues, and how might this innervation contribute to the photoperiod/MEL affects on these tissues?

Sympathetic Nervous System and Photoperiodic Body and Lipid Mass Cycles

Both BAT[82] and WAT[140] are innervated by the sympathetic nervous system. The innervation of BAT by the SNS is undisputed and has been known for over 30 years.[141] *Functional* evidence for the SNS innervation of WAT has been accumulating for nearly 85 years.[142] Controversy has existed concerning the *neuroanatomical* evidence for the SNS innervation of WAT until recently, even though the initial report of the SN innervation of WAT was made over 100 years ago.[143] The first neuroanatomical evidence of direct SNS innervation of WAT was demonstrated using retrograde and anterograde tract tracing methodologies recently.[144] Briefly, we found that the IWAT and EWAT pads of Siberian hamsters are innervated relatively separately by postganglionic neurons in the sympathetic chain. This study was prompted by an earlier finding reporting a non-uniform pattern of lipid mobilization from SD-exposed Siberian hamsters.[119] Specifically, the more internally located pads show the greatest lipid mobilization after SD exposure, and the more externally located pads show the least lipid mobilization after SD exposure.[67,72,119,145] The separate neuroanatomical pattern of post ganglionic, SNS innervation of WAT pads made it possible anatomically that the SD-induced differential rate of lipid depletion in these pads could be due to different SNS neural drives on the internal vs. externally located WAT pads. Indeed, norepinephrine turnover, an indicator of SNS drive,[146] was greater in EWAT mass than in IWAT, corresponding to the greater decrease in EWAT than IWAT mass after SD exposure in Siberian hamsters.[144]

The neuroanatomical substrate for the innervation of the SNS outflow from the brain to WAT and BAT has been defined recently using transneuronal viral tract tracers in Siberian hamsters and laboratory rats.[80,81] An attenuated strain of the pseudorabies virus, Bartha's K strain, was used. Briefly, the virus is taken up into neurons following binding to viral attachment protein molecules found on the surface of neuronal membranes. These protein surface molecules act as "viral receptors". Neurons synapsing on infected cells become exposed to relatively high concentrations of the virus particles that have been exocytosed. The virus particles are then taken up by synaptic contact. This process continues causing an infection along the neuronal chain from the periphery to higher CNS sites.[147,148] The virus is then visualized using standard immunocytochemical methods.

Application of this viral technology to the study of the innervation of WAT and BAT has revealed more similarities than differences in the CNS origins of the SNS outflow from brain to these two adipose tissue types.[80,81] Specifically, infected cells occur at all levels of the neuroaxis for both adipose tissue types and include: (1) the sympathetic chain, (2) the spinal cord (intermediolateral cell column, central autonomic nucleus), (3) the brainstem (intermediate reticular nucleus, gigantocelluar reticular nucleus, caudal raphe nucleus, C1 adrenaline and A5 noradrenaline cell regions, nucleus of the solitary tract), (4) the midbrain (central gray), and (5) the forebrain (paraventricular, lateral, dorsomedial and suprachiasmatic hypothalamic nuclei, medial preoptic area, arcuate nucleus, bed nucleus of the stria terminalis, lateral septum). Thus, any or all of these areas could be involved in the photoperiod/ MEL modulation of WAT and BAT in this and other species. A beginning toward answering which of these areas might be involved in these photoperiodic responses awaits the results of studies in progress, in which co-localization of CNS sympathetic neurons, as revealed through pseudorabies tract tracing studies with neurons producing Mel-1a receptor mRNA, will be sought.

Summary

We have reviewed possible hormonal intermediaries that result in the effects of the photoperiod/MEL on energy balance, especially changes in WAT lipid accumulation or mobilization. This was done for several species of small rodents that demonstrate seasonal reproductive cycles controlled by the photoperiod/MEL. To date, none of the hormones examined appears to be a likely candidate for the role of the intermediary agent for the effects of the photoperiod/MEL on the level of adiposity. One possible hormonal candidate that deserves more study is glucagon. Finally, the possible role of the SNS innervation of WAT and BAT was discussed as a means by which the photoperiod/MEL could affect these adipose tissues.

Acknowledgments

The authors thank Drs. Maryam Bamshad and Gregory Demas for their comments on this review, and especially Dr. George Wade for his role in shaping this area of investigation and the career of the senior author.

This work was supported in part by the National Institutes of Health RO1 DK35254 & RO1 DK47246, and National Institute of Mental Health Research Scientist Development Award KO2 MH00841 to TJB.

References

1. Rodin, J., Psychological factors in obesity, in Bjorntorp, P., Cairella, M., and Howard, A.N., Eds., *Recent Advances in Obesity Research, III,* John Libbey, London, 1981, 106.

2. Sclafani, A., Animal models of obesity: classification and characterization, *Int. J. Obesity,* 8, 491–508, 1984.

3. Mrosovsky, N. and Barnes, D., Anorexia, food deprivation and hibernation, *Physiol. Behav.,* 12, 265–270, 1974.

4. Bartness, T.J. and Wade, G.N., Seasonal body weight cycles in hamsters, *Neurosci. Biobehav. Rev.,* 9, 599–612, 1985.

5. Mrosovsky, N., Body fat during pregnancy and lactation, in Cioffi, L.A., Ed., *The Body Weight Regulatory System: Normal and Disturbed Mechanisms,* Raven Press, New York, 1981, 253.

6. Bronson, F.H., Heideman, P.D., and Kerbeshian, M.C., Lability of fat stores in peripubertal wild house mice, *J. Comp. Physiol. B,* 161, 15–18, 1991.

7. Rusak, B., Mistlerger, R.E., Losier, B., and Jones, C.H., Daily hoarding opportunity entrains the pacemaker for hamster activity rhythms, *J. Comp. Physiol. A,* 164, 165–171, 1988.

8. Young, R.A., Salans, L.B., and Sims, E.A.H., Adipose tissue cellularity in woodchucks: effects of season and captivity at an early age, *J. Lipid Res.,* 23, 887–892, 1988.

9. Dark, J., Stern, J.S., and Zucker, I., Adipose tissue dynamics during cyclic weight loss and weight gain of ground squirrels, *Am. J. Physiol.,* 256, R1286–R1292, 1989.

10. Bartness, T.J., Powers, J.B., Hastings, M.H., Bittman, E.L., and Goldman, B.D., The timed infusion paradigm for melatonin delivery: what has it taught us about the melatonin signal, its reception and the photoperiodic control of seasonal responses?, *J. Pineal Res.,* 15, 161–190, 1993.

11. Bartness, T.J. and Goldman, B.D., Mammalian pineal melatonin: a clock for all seasons, *Experientia*, 45, 939–945, 1989.

12. Bjorntorp, P., Adipose tissue distribution and function. *Int. J. Obesity*, 15, 67–81, 1991.

13. Himms-Hagen, J., Brown adipose tissue metabolism and thermogenesis, *Ann. Rev. Nutr.*, 5, 69–94, 1985.

14. Turek, F.W. and Campbell, C.S., Photoperiodic regulation of neuroendocrine-gonadal activity, *Biol. Reprod.*, 20, 32–50, 1979.

15. Bronson, F.H. and Heideman, P.D., Seasonal regulation of reproduction in mammals, in Knobil, E. and Neill, J.D., Eds., *The Physiology of Reproduction*, Second ed., Raven Press, New York, 1994, 541.

16. Underwood, H. and Goldman, B.D., Vertebrate circadian and photoperiodic systems: role of the pineal gland and melatonin, *J. Biol. Rhythms*, 2, 279–315, 1987.

17. Stetson, M.H. and Watson-Whitmyre, M., The physiology of the pineal and its hormone melatonin in annual reproduction in rodents, in Reiter, R.J.R., Ed., *The Pineal Gland*, Raven Press, New York, 1984, 109.

18. Moore, R.Y., Neural control of the pineal gland, *Behav. Brain Res.*, 73, 125–130, 1996.

19. Bartness, T.J. and Wade, G.N., Photoperiodic control of body weight and energy metabolism in Syrian hamsters (*Mesocricetus auratus*): role of pineal gland, melatonin, gonads and diet, *Endocrinology*, 114, 492–498, 1984.

20. Hoffman, R.A., Seasonal growth and development and the influence of the eyes and pineal gland on body weight of golden hamsters (*M. auratus*), *Growth*, 47, 109–121, 1983.

21. Vitale, P.M., Darrow, J.M., Duncan, M.J., Shustak, C.A., and Goldman, B.D., Effects of photoperiod, pinealectomy and castration on body weight and daily torpor in Djungarian hamsters (*Phodopus sungorus*), *J. Endocrinol.*, 106, 367–375, 1985.

22. Bartness, T.J. and Goldman, B.D., Peak duration of serum melatonin and short day responses in adult Siberian hamsters, *Am. J. Physiol.*, 255, R812–R822, 1988.

23. Bartness, T.J. and Goldman, B.D., Effects of melatonin on long day responses in short day-housed adult Siberian hamsters, *Am. J. Physiol.*, 255, R823-R830, 1988.

24. Rhodes, D.H., The influence of multiple photoperiods and pinealectomy on gonads, pelage and body weight in male meadow voles, *Microtus pennsylvanicus*, *Comp. Biochem. Physiol. A*, 93, 445–449, 1989.

25. Smale, L., Dark, J., and Zucker, I., Pineal and photoperiodic influences on fat deposition, pelage, and testicular activity in male meadow voles, *J. Biol. Rhythms*, 3, 349–355, 1988.

26. Hastings, M.H., Neuroendocrine rhythms, *Pharmaceut. Ther.*, 50, 35–71, 1991.

27. Elliott, J.A. and Goldman, B.D., Seasonal reproduction, photoperiodism and biological clocks, in Adler, N.T., Ed., *Neuroendocrinology of Reproduction*, Plenum Press, New York, 1981, 377.

28. Tamarkin, L., Westrom, W.K., Hamill, A.I., and Goldman, B.D., Effect of melatonin on the reproductive systems of male and female hamsters: a diurnal rhythm in sensitivity to melatonin, *Endocrinology,* 99, 1534–1541, 1976.

29. Maywood, E.S., Hastings, M.H., Max, M., Ampleford, E., Menaker, M., and Loudon, A.S.I., Circadian and daily rhythms of melatonin in the blood and pineal gland of free-running and entrained Syrian hamsters, *J. Endocrinol.,* 136, 65–73, 1993.

30. Brown, G.M., Seggie, J., and Grota, L.J., Serum melatonin response to melatonin administration in the Syrian hamster, *Neuroendocrinology,* 41, 31–35, 1985.

31. Song, C.K. and Bartness, T.J., Microknife-cuts dorsal and caudal to the suprachiasmatic nucleus do not block short day responses by Siberian hamsters to timed infusions of melatonin, *Brain Res. Bull.,* 45, 239–246, 1998.

32. Song, C.K. and Bartness, T.J., The effects of anterior hypothalamic lesions on short day responses in Siberian hamsters given timed infusions of melatonin, *J. Biol. Rhythms,* 11, 14–26, 1996.

33. Bittman, E.L., The sites and consequences of melatonin binding in mammals, *Am. Zool.,* 33, 200–211, 1993.

34. Weaver, D.R., Rivkees, S.A., Carlson, L.L., and Reppert, S.M., Localization of melatonin receptors in mammalian brain, in Klein, D.C., Moore, R.Y., and Reppert, S.M., Eds., *Suprachiasmatic Nucleus: The Mind's Clock,* Oxford University Press, New York, 1991, 289.

35. Morgan, P.J., Barrett, P., Howell, E., and Helliwell, R., Melatonin receptors: localizaton, molecular pharmacology and physiological significance, *Neurochem. Int.,* 24, 101–146, 1994.

36. Bittman, E.L. and Weaver, D.R., Distribution of melatonin receptors in neuroendo-crine tissues of the ewe, *Biol. Reprod.,* 43, 986–993, 1990.

37. Duncan, M.J., Takahashi, J.S., and Dubocovich, M.L., Characteristics and autoradio-graphic localization of 2-[^{125}I]iodomelatonin binding sites in Djungarian hamster brain, *Endocrinology,* 125, 1011–1018, 1989.

38. Williams, L.M., Morgan, P.J., Hastings, M.H., Lawson, W., Davidson, G., and Howell, H.E., Melatonin receptor sites in the Syrian hamster brain and pituitary. Localization and characterization using [^{125}I]iodomelatonin, *J. Neuroendocrinol.,* 1, 315–320, 1989.

39. Reppert, S.M., Weaver, D.R., Rivkees, S.A., and Stopa, E.G., Putative melatonin receptors in a human biological clock, *Science,* 242, 78–81, 1988.

40. Duncan, M.J. and Mead, R.A., Autoradiographic localization of binding sites for 2-[^{125}I]iodomelatonin in the pars tuberalis of the western spotted skunk (*Spilogale putorius latifrons*), *Brain Res.,* 569, 152–155, 1992.

41. Weaver, D.R. and Reppert, S.M., Melatonin receptors are present in the ferret pars tuberalis and pars distalis, but not in brain, *Endocrinology,* 127, 2607–2609, 1990.

42. Reppert, S.M., Weaver, D.R., and Ebisawa, T., Cloning and characterization of a mammalian melatonin receptor that mediates reproductive and circadian responses, *Neuron,* 13, 1177–1185, 1994.

43. Bartness, T.J., Goldman, B.D., and Bittman, E.L., SCN lesions block responses to peripheral melatonin infusions in Siberian hamsters, *Am. J. Physiol.,* 260, R102–R112, 1991.

44. Maywood, E.S., Buttery, R.C., Vance, G.H.S., Herbert, J., and Hastings, M.H., Gonadal responses of the male Syrian hamster to programmed infusions of melatonin are sensitive to signal duration and frequency but not to signal phase nor to lesions of the suprachiasmatic nuclei, *Biol. Reprod.,* 43, 174–182, 1990.

45. Ng, T.B. and Wong, C.M., Effects of pineal indoles and arginine vasotocin on lipolysis and lipogenesis in isolated adipocytes, *J. Pineal Res.,* 3, 55–66, 1986.

46. Hoffman, R.A., Hester, R.J., and Towns, C., Effect of light and temperature on the endocrine system of the golden hamster (*Mesocricetus auratus* Waterhouse), *Comp. Biochem. Physiol.,* 15, 525–535, 1965.

47. Canguilhem, B., Vaultier, J.-P., Pevet, P., Coumaros, G., Masson-Pevet, M., and Bentz, I., Photoperiodic regulation of body mass, food intake, hibernation, and reproduction in intact and castrated European hamsters, *Cricetus cricetus, J. Comp. Physiol. A,* 163, 549–557, 1988.

48. Figala, J., Hoffmann, K., and Goldau, G., Zur Jahresperiodik beim Dsungarischen Zwerghamster *Phodopus sungorus* Pallas, *Oecologia,* 12, 89–118, 1973.

49. Hoffmann, K., The influence of photoperiod and melatonin on testis size, body weight and pelage colour in the Djungarian hamster (*Phodopus sungorus*), *J. Comp. Physiol.,* 85, 267–282, 1973.

50. Nelson, R.J., Frank, D., Smale, L., and Willoughby, S.B., Photoperiod and temperature affect reproductive and nonreproductive functions in male prairie voles (*Microtus ochrogaster*), *Biol. Reprod.,* 40, 481–485, 1989.

51. Dark, J., Zucker, I., and Wade, G.N., Photoperiodic regulation of body mass, food intake, and reproduction in meadow voles, *Am. J. Physiol.,* 245, R334–R338, 1983.

52. Hasler, J.F., Buhl, A.E., and Banks, E.M., The influence of photoperiod on growth and sexual function in male and female collared lemmings, *J. Reprod. Fert.,* 46, 323–329, 1976.

53. Dark, J., Johnston, P.G., Healy, M., and Zucker, I., Latitude of origin influences photoperiodic control of reproduction of deer mice (*Peromyscus maniculatus*), *Biol. Reprod.,* 28, 213–220, 1983.

54. Whitsett, J.M., Underwood, H., and Cherry, J., Photoperiodic stimulation of pubertal development in male deer mice: involvement of the circadian system, *Biol. Reprod.,* 28, 652–656, 1983.

55. Gower, B.A., Nagy, T.R., and Stetson, M.H., Effect of photoperiod, testosterone, and estradiol on body mass, bifid claw size and pelage color in collared lemmings, *Gen. Comp. Endocrinol.,* 93, 459–470, 1994.

56. Kriegsfeld, L.J. and Nelson, R.J., Gonadal and photoperiodic influences on body mass regulation in adult male and female prairie voles, *Am. J. Physiol. Regul. Integr. Comp. Physiol.,* 270, R1013–R1018, 1996.

57. Hoffman, R.A., Davidson, K., and Steinberg, K., Influence of photoperiod and temperature on weight gain, food consumption, fat pads and thyroxine in male golden hamsters, *Growth,* 46, 150–162, 1982.

58. Campbell, C.S., Tabor, J., and Davis, J.D., Small effect of brown adipose tissue and major effect of photoperiod on body weight in hamsters (*Mesocricetus auratus*), *Physiol. Behav.,* 30, 349–352, 1983.

59. Flint, W.E., *Die Zwerghamster der Palaarktischen Fauna,* Ziemse-Verlag, Wittenberg Lutherstadt, FRG, 1966.

60. Steinlechner, S., Heldmaier, G., and Becker, H., The seasonal cycle of body weight in the Djungarian hamster: photoperiodic control and the influence of starvation and melatonin, *Oecologia,* 60, 401–405, 1983.

61. Wade, G.N. and Bartness, T.J., Effects of photoperiod and gonadectomy on food intake, body weight and body composition in Siberian hamsters, *Am. J. Physiol.,* 246, R26–R30, 1984.

62. Dark, J. and Zucker, I., Gonadal and photoperiodic control of seasonal body weight changes in male voles, *Am. J. Physiol.,* 247, R84–R88, 1984.

63. Nelson, R.J., Kita, M., Blom, J.M., and Rhyne-Grey, J., Photoperiod influences the critical caloric intake necessary to maintain reproduction among male deer mice (*Peromyscus maniculatus*), *Biol. Reprod.,* 46, 226–232, 1992.

64. Blank, J.L., Korytko, A.I., Freeman, D.A., and Ruf, T.P., Role of gonadal steroid and inhibitory photoperiod in regulating body weight and food intake in deer mice (*Peromyscus maniculatus*), *Proc. Soc. Exp. Biol. Med.,* 206, 396–403, 1994.

65. Morin, L.P. and Fleming, A., Variations of food intake and body weight with estrous cycle, ovariectomy, and estradiol benzoate treatment in hamsters (*Mesocriceuts auratus*), *J. Comp. Physiol. Psychol.,* 92, 1–6, 1976.

66. Slusser, W.N. and Wade, G.N., Testicular effects on food intake, body weight and body composition in male hamsters, *Physiol. Behav.,* 27, 637–640, 1981.

67. Bartness, T.J., Photoperiod, sex, gonadal steroids and housing density affect body fat in hamsters, *Physiol. Behav.,* 60, 517–529, 1996.

68. Blank, J.L. and Freeman, D.A., Differential reproductive response to short photoperiod in deer mice: role of melatonin, *J. Comp. Physiol.,* 169, 501–506, 1991.

69. Dark, J., Whaling, C.S., and Zucker, I., Androgens exert opposite effects on body mass of heavy and light meadow voles, *Horm. Behav.,* 21, 471–477, 1987.

70. Canguilhem, B., Masson-Pevet, M., Pevet, P., and Bentz, I., Endogenous, photoperiodic and hormonal control of the body weight rhythm in the female European hamster, *Cricetus cricetus, Comp. Biochem. Physiol. Comp. Physiol.,* 101, 465–470, 1992.

71. Dark, J. and Zucker, I., Photoperiodic regulation of body mass and fat reserves in the meadow vole, *Physiol. Behav.,* 38, 851–854, 1986.

72. Bartness, T.J., Short day-induced depletion of lipid stores is fat pad- and gender-specific in Siberian hamsters, *Physiol. Behav.,* 58, 539–550, 1995.

73. Bartness, T.J., Elliott, J.A., and Goldman, B.D., Control of torpor and body weight patterns by a seasonal timer in Siberian hamsters, *Am. J. Physiol.,* 257, R142–R149, 1989.

74. Wade, G.N. and Bartness, T.J., Seasonal obesity in Syrian hamsters: effects of age, diet, photoperiod, and melatonin, *Am. J. Physiol.,* 247, R328–R334, 1984.

75. Hoffmann, K., Effect of castration on photoperiodically induced weight gain in the Djungarian hamster, *Naturwissenschaften* 65, 494, 1978.

76. Saulnier-Blache, J.-S., Larrouy, D., Carpene, C., Quideau, N., Dauzats, M., and Lafontan, M., Photoperiodic control of adipocyte alpha2-adrenoceptors in Syrian hamsters: role of testosterone, *Endocrinology,* 127, 1245–1253, 1990.

77. Carpene, C., Berlan, M., and Lafontan, M., Lack of functional antilipolytic alpha2-adrenoceptor in rat fat cell: comparison with hamster adipocyte, *Comp. Biochem. Physiol.,* 74C, 41–45, 1983.

78. Bouloumie, A., Valet, P., Daviaud, D., Prats, H., Lafontan, M., and Saulnier-Blache, J.-S., Adipocyte α_{2A}-adrenoceptor is the only α_2-adrenoceptor regulated by testosterone, *Eur. J. Pharmacol.,* 269, 95–103, 1995.

79. Bouloumie, A., Valet, P., Dauzats, M., Lafontan, M., and Saulnier-Blache, J.-S., *In vivo* upregulation of adipocyte α_2-adrenoceptors by androgens is consequence of direct action on fat cells, *Am. J. Physiol.,* 267, C926–C931, 1994.

80. Bamshad, M. and Bartness, T.J., Central nervous system origins of the sympathetic nervous system outflow to brown adipose tissue, *Am. J. Physiol.* (in press).

81. Bamshad, M., Aoki, V.T., Adkison, M.G., Warren, W.S., and Bartness, T.J., Central nervous system origins of the sympathetic nervous system outflow to white adipose tissue, *Am. J. Physiol.,* 275, R291–R299, 1998.

82. Bartness, T.J. and Bamshad, M., Innervation of mammalian white adipose tissue: implications for the regulation of total body fat, *Am. J. Physiol.* (in press).

83. Agius, L., Robinson, A.M., Girard, J.R., and Williamson, D.H., Alterations in the rate of lipogenesis *in vivo* in maternal liver and adipose tissue on premature weaning of lactating rats, *Biochem. J.,* 180, 689–692, 1979.

84. Smith, R.W., Effect of pregnancy, lactation and involution on metabolism of glucose by rat parametrial adipose tissue, *J. Dairy Res.,* 40, 353–360, 1973.

85. Ortavant, R., Bocquier, F., Pelletier, J., Ravault, J.P., Thimonier, J., and Volland-Nail, P., Seasonality of reproduction in sheep and its control by photoperiod, *Aust. J. Biol. Sci.,* 41, 69–85, 1988.

86. Goldman, B.D., Matt, K.S., Roychoudhury, P., and Stetson, M.H., Prolactin release in golden hamsters: photoperiod and gonadal influences, *Biol. Reprod.,* 24, 287–292, 1981.

87. Borer, K.T., Kelch, R.P., and Corley, K., Hamster prolactin: physiological changes in blood and pituitary concentrations as measured by a homologous radioimmunoassay, *Neuroendocrinology,* 35, 12–21, 1982.

88. Yellon, S.M. and Goldman, B.D., Influence of short days on diurnal patterns of serum gonadotrophins and prolactin concentrations in the male Djungarian hamster, *Phodopus sungorus, J. Reprod. Fert.,* 80, 167–174, 1987.

89. Whitten, R.D., Youngstrom, T.G., and Bartness, T.J., Hyperprolactinemia does not promote testicular recrudescence in photoregressed Siberian hamsters, *Physiol. Behav.,* 54, 175–178, 1993.

90. Bartness, T.J., Wade, G.N., and Goldman, B.D., Are the short photoperiod decreases in serum prolactin responsible for the seasonal changes in energy balance in Syrian and Siberian hamsters?, *J. Exp. Zool.*, 244, 437–454, 1987.

91. Duncan, M.J. and Goldman, B.D., Hormonal regulation of the annual pelage cycle in the Djungarian hamster, *Phodopus sungorus*. II. Role of prolactin, *J. Exp. Zool.*, 230, 97–103, 1984.

92. Duncan, M.J. and Goldman, B.D., Physiological doses of prolactin stimulate pelage pigmentation in Djungarian hamster, *Am. J. Physiol.*, 248, R664–R667, 1985.

93. Cincotta, A.H. and Meier, A.H., Reduction of body fat stores by inhibition of prolactin secretion, *Experientia*, 43, 416–417, 1985.

94. Cincotta, A.H., MacEachern, T.A., and Meier, A.H., Bromocriptine redirects metabolism and prevents seasonal onset of obese hyerinsulinemic state in Syrian hamsters, *Am. J. Physiol.*, 264, E285–E293, 1993.

95. Cincotta, A.H., Schiller, B.C., and Meier, A.H., Bromocryptine inhibits the seasonally occurring obesity, hyperinsulinemia, insulin resistance, and impaired glucose tolerance in the Syrian hamster, *Mesocricetus auratus, Metabolism*, 40, 639–644, 1991.

96. Cincotta, A.H. and Meier, A.H., Bromocryptine inhibits *in vivo* free fatty acid oxidation and hepatic glucose output in seasonally obese hamsters (*Mesocricetus auratus*), *Metabolism*, 44, 1349–1355, 1995.

97. Cincotta, A.H., Wilson, J.M., deSouza, C.J., and Meier, A.H., Properly timed injections of cortisol and prolactin produce long-term reductions in obesity, hyperinsulinaemia and insulin resistance in the Syrian hamster (*Mesocrietus auratus*), *J. Endocrinol.*, 120, 385–391, 1989.

98. Collins, S., Kuhn, C.M., Petro, A.E., Swick, A.G., Chrunyk, B.A., and Surwit, R.S., Role of leptin in fat regulation, *Nature*, 380, 677–677, 1996.

99. Kott, K.S., Moore, B.J., Fournier, L., and Horwitz, B.A., Hyperprolactinemia prevents short photoperiod-induced changes in brown fat, *Am. J. Physiol.*, 256, R174–R180, 1989.

100. Vriend, J., Evidence for pineal gland modulation of the neuroendocrine-thyroid axis, *Neuroendocrinology*, 36, 68–78, 1983.

101. Vriend, J.B., Richardson, B.A., Vaughan, M.K., Johnson, L.Y., and Reiter, R.J.R., Effects of melatonin on thyroid physiology of female hamsters, *Neuroendocrinology*, 35, 79–85, 1982.

102. Ottenweller, J.E., Tapp, W.N., Pittman, D.L., and Natelson, B.H., Adrenal, thyroid, and testicular hormone rhythms in male golden hamsters on long and short days, *Am. J. Physiol.*, 253, R321–R328, 1987.

103. Nagy, T.R., Gower, B.A., and Stetson, M.H., Photoperiod effects on body mass, body composition, growth hormone, and thyroid hormones in male collared lemmings (*Dicrostonyx groenlandicus*), *Can. J. Zool.*, 72, 1726–1734, 1994.

104. Nagy, T.R., Gower, B.A., and Stetson, M.H., Endocrine correlates of seasonal body mass dynamics in the collared lemming (*Dicrostonyx groenlandicus*), *Am. Zool.*, 35, 246–258, 1995.

105. Seidel, A., Heldmaier, G., and Schulz, F., Seasonal changes in circulating levels of thyroid hormones are not dependent on the age in Djungarian hamsters *Phodopus sungorus*, *Comp. Biochem. Physiol.*, 88*A*, 71–73, 1987.

106. Masuda, A. and Oishi, T., Effects of photoperiod, temperature and testosterone-treatment on plasma T_3 and T_4 levels in the Djungarian hamster, *Phodopus sungorus*, *Experientia*, 45, 102–103, 1989.

107. O'Jile, J.R. and Bartness, T.J., Effects of thyroxine on the photoperiodic control of energy balance and reproductive status in Siberian hamsters, *Physiol. Behav.*, 52, 267–270, 1992.

108. Zoeller, R.T., Kabeer, N., and Albers, H.E., Cold exposure elevates cellular levels of mRNA encoding thyrotropin-releasing hormone (TRH) in paraventricular nucleus despite elevated levels of thyroid hormones, *Endocrinology*, 127, 2955–2962, 1990.

109. Bray, G.A. and York, D.A., Hypothalamic and genetic obesity in experimental animals: an autonomic and endocrine hypothesis, *J. Physiol.*, 377, 1–13, 1979.

110. Ottenweller, J.E., Tapp, W.N., Burke, J.M., and Natelson, B.H., Plasma cortisol and corticosterone concentrations in the golden hamster (*Mesocricetus auratus*), *Life Sci.*, 37, 1551–1558, 1985.

111. Williams, K.A., Role of Glucocorticoids in the Photoperiodic Control of Body Weight, Body Fat and Food Intake in Siberian Hamsters, unpublished Masters thesis, Georgia State University, 1994.

112. Nelson, R.J., Fine, J.B., Demas, G.E., and Moffatt, C.A., Photoperiod and population density interact to affect reproductive and immune function in male prairie voles, *Am. J. Physiol. Regul. Integr. Comp. Physiol.*, 270, R571–R577, 1996.

113. Fischman, A.J., Kastin, A.J., Graf, M.V., and Moldow, R.L., Constant light and dark affect the circadian rhythm of the hypothalamic-pituitary-adrenal axis, *Neuroendocrinology*, 47, 309–316, 1988.

114. Allen-Rowlands, C.F., Allen, J.P., Greer, M.A., and Wilson, M., Circadian rhythmicity of ACTH and corticosterone in the rat, *J. Endocrinol. Invest.*, 3, 371–377, 1980.

115. Veldhuis, J.D., Iranmanesh, A., Lizarralde, G., and Johnson, M.L., Amplitude modulation of a burstlike mode of cortisol secretion subserves the circadian glucocorticoid rhythm, *Am. J. Physiol.*, 257, E6–E14, 1989.

116. Bartness, T.J., McGriff, W.R., Maharaj, M.P., and Borer, K.T., Photoperiodic control of serum insulin: effects on energy balance and reproductive status in Siberian hamsters (abstract), *FASEB Abstr.*, 1991.

117. Feldman, D. and Loose, D., Glucocorticoid receptors in adipose tissue, *Endocrinology*, 100, 398–405, 1977.

118. Gray, G.O. and Leavitt, W.W., RU486 is not an antiprogestin in the hamster, *J. Steroid Biochem.*, 28, 493–497, 1987.

119. Bartness, T.J., Hamilton, J.M., Wade, G.N., and Goldman, B.D., Regional differences in fat pad responses to short days in Siberian hamsters, *Am. J. Physiol.*, 257, R1533–R1540, 1989.

120. Langley, S.C. and York, D.A., Effects of antiglucocorticoid RU486 on development of obesity in obese fa/fa Zucker rats, *Am. J. Physiol.*, 259, R539–R544, 1990.

121. Okada, S., York, D.A., and Bray, G.A., Mifepristone (RU486), a blocker of type II glucocorticoid and progestin receptors, reverses a dietary form of obesity, *Am. J. Physiol.*, 262, R1106–R1110, 1992.

122. Miceli, M.O., Post, C.A., and Woshowska, Z., Abdominal vagotomy blocks hyperphagia and body weight gain in Syrian hamsters exposed to short photoperiod (abstract), Society for Neuroscience Meeting Abstract 522.4, 1989.

123. Schwartz, M.W., Figelwicz, D.P., Baskin, D.G., Woods, S.C., and Porte, Jr., D., Insulin: a hormonal regulator of energy balance, *Endocrine Rev.*, 13, 387–414, 1992.

124. Woods, S.C. and Porte, Jr., D., Insulin and the set-point regulation of body weight, in *Hunger: Basic Mechanisms and Clinical Implications*, Raven Press, New York, 1976, 273.

125. Bartness, T.J., McGriff, W.R., and Maharaj, M.P., Effect of diabetes and insulin on photoperiodic responses in Siberian hamsters, *Physiol. Behav.*, 49, 613-620, 1991.

126. LeMagnen, J., Metabolic and feeding patterns: role of sympathetic and parasympathetic efferent pathways, *J. Auton. Nerv. Syst.*, 10, 325–335, 1984.

127. Borer, K.T., Kelch, R.P., and Hayashida, T., Hamster growth hormone. Species specifity and physiological changes in blood and pituitary, *Neuroendocrinology*, 35, 349, 1982.

128. Vriend, J., Borer, K.T., and Thilveris, J.A., Melatonin: its antagonism of thyroxine's antisomatotrophic activity in male Syrian hamsters, *Growth* 51, 35–43, 1987.

129. Vriend, J., Sheppard, M.S., and Borer, K.T., Melatonin increases serum growth hormone and insulin-like growth factorI (IGF-I) levels in male Syrian hamsters via hypothalamic neurotransmitters, *Growth Dev. Aging*, 54, 165–171, 1990.

130. Peter, M.A., Winterhalter, K.H., Boni-Schnetzler, M., Froesch, E.R., and Zapf, J., Regulation of insulin-like growth factor-I (IGF-I) and IGF-binding proteins by growth hormone in rat white adipose tissue, *Endocrinology*, 133, 2524–2631, 1993.

131. Bjorntorp, P., Growth hormone, insulin-like growth factor-I and lipid metabolism: interactions with sex steroids, *Horm. Res.*, 46, 188–191, 1996.

132. Wabitsch, M., Hauner, H., Heinze, E., and Teller, W.M., The role of growth hormone/insulin-like growth factors in adipocyte differentiation, *Metabolism* 44, 45–49, 1995.

133. Nougues, J., Reyne, Y., Barenton, B., Chery, T., Garandel, V., and Soriano, J., Differentiation of adipocyte precursors in a serum-free medium is influenced by glucocorticoids and endogenously produced insulin-like growth factor-I, *Int. J. Obesity*, 17, 159–167, 1993.

134. Wade, G.N., Dietary obesity in golden hamsters: reversibility and effects of sex and photoperiod, *Physiol. Behav.*, 30, 131–137, 1983.

135. Vriend, J., Sheppard, M.S., and Bala, R.M., Melatonin increases serum insulin-like growth factor-I in male Syrian hamsters, *Endocrinology*, 122, 2558–2561, 1988.

136. Billington, C.J., Briggs, J.E., Link, J.G., and Levine, A.S., Glucagon in physiological concentrations stimulates brown fat thermogenesis *in vivo*, *Am. J. Physiol.*, 261, R501–R507, 1991.

137.   Yahata, T. and Kuroshima, A., Metabolic cold acclimation after repetitive intermittent cold exposure in rat, *Jpn. J. Physiol.,* 39, 215–228, 1989.

138.   Iwanij, V., Amos, T.M., and Billington, C.J., Identification and characterization of the glucagon receptor from adipose tissue, *Mol. Cell. Endocrinol.,* 101, 257–261, 1994.

139.   Billington, C.J., Bartness, T.J., Briggs, J., Levine, A.S., and Morley, J.E., Glucagon stimulation of brown adipose tissue growth and thermogenesis, *Am. J. Physiol.,* 252, R160–R165, 1987.

140.   Himms-Hagen, J., Neural control of brown adipose tissue thermogenesis, hypertrophy, and atrophy, *Frontiers Neuroendocrinol.,* 12, 38–93, 1991.

141.   Wirsen, C., Studies in lipid mobilization with special reference to morphological and histochemical aspects, *Acta Physiol. Scand.,* 65, 1–46, 1965.

142.   Mansfeld, G. and Muller, F., Der Einfluss der Nervensystem auf die Mobilisierung von Fett, *Arch. Physiol.,* 152, 61–67, 1913.

143.   Dogiel, A.S., Die sensiblen Nervenendigungen im Herzen und in den Blutgefassen der Saugethiere, *Arch. Mikr. Anat.,* 52, 44–70, 1898.

144.   Youngstrom, T.G. and Bartness, T.J., Catecholaminergic innervation of white adipose tissue in the Siberian hamster, *Am. J. Physiol.,* 268, R744–R751, 1995.

145.   Bartness, T.J. and Wade, G.N., Effects of interscapular brown adipose tissue denervation on estrogen-induced changes in food intake, body weight and energy metabolism, *Behav. Neurosci.,* 98, 674–685, 1984.

146.   Young, J.B. and Landsberg, L., Suppression of the sympathetic nervous system during fasting, *Science,* 196, 1473–1475, 1977.

147.   Jansen, A.S.P., Farwell, D.G., and Loewy, A.D., Specificity of pseudorabies virus as a retrograde marker of sympathetic preganglionic neurons: implications for transneuronal labeling studies, *Brain Res.,* 617, 103–112, 1993.

148.   Strack, A.M. and Loewy, A.D, Pseudorabies virus: a highly specific transneuronal cell body marker in the sympathetic nervous system, *J. Neurosci.,* 10, 2139–2147, 1990.

Chapter 8

Pineal Gland Neuropeptides

Bryant Benson

Contents

Introduction

It is well established that a polysynaptic pathway conveys information about light from the retina to the pineal gland with relays in the suprachiasmatic and paraventricular nuclei of the hypothalamus, the spinal cord, and superior cervical ganglia.[1,2] The post-ganglionic sympathetic fibers innervating the pineal[3] provide nocturnal activation of melatonin secretion via β_1- and α_1-adrenergic cAMP-dependent activation of N-acetyltransferase (NAT), the rate-limiting enzyme for melatonin synthesis.[4] Yet, other neurotransmitters and their receptors have been localized to the pineals of several mammals,[5,6] and the observation that factors other than light can modulate peak melatonin secretion[7] suggests that more than one transmitter may be involved in the regulation of indoleamine synthesis.[8,9] This idea is reinforced by the observation that neural connections exist between the pineal gland and specific portions of the central and parasympathetic nervous systems.[10–12]

Over the last two decades, specific antibodies to neuropeptides of known structure have been developed and applied in immunocytochemical studies of mammalian pineal glands. A partial list of neuropeptides identified by this or other methods is presented in Table 1. For the most part, the function of these pineal neuropeptides is unknown, although many were observed in pinealopetal nerve fibers and are postulated to modulate pinealocyte melatonin synthesis and release.

Neuropeptide Y

One neuropeptide studied most extensively is neuropeptide Y (NPY), a 36-amino-acid polypeptide found abundantly in various portions of the mammalian nervous system, including the pineal gland.[12] NPY is often co-localized with catecholamines and may be involved in the regulation of important physiological functions such as vasoconstriction, hormone synthesis and release, food and water intake, and certain learning behaviors. The pineal glands of all mammals studied have been shown to possess NPY innervation, only part of which is lost after bilateral superior cervical ganglionectomy depending on the species.[12,13] Extra sympathetic NPY innervation probably originates from the intergeniculate leaflet of the lateral geniculate body which contains a high density of NPY neurons.[14] Anterograde tracing studies in the rat and gerbil have shown a direct connection between this structure and the pineal gland,[15,16] suggesting that a visual input may come more directly to the pineal gland than previously thought.

NYP was shown by Vacas et al.[17] and Simonneaux et al.[18] to inhibit up to 45% of the presynaptic release of pineal NE ($EC_{50} = 50$ nM) through NPY-Y2 receptors. Incubated with dissociated pinealocytes *in vitro*, NPY induced a weak postsynaptic inhibition of norepinephrine (NE)- or vasoactive intestinal peptide (VIP)-induced stimulation of cAMP via NPY-Y1 receptors.[18–20]

While these inhibitory effects of NYP on NE are well documented, effects on melatonin synthesis and release are diversely reported to be either inhibitory or moderately stimulatory, depending on the investigator and systems utilized.[17,18,20,21] Because scotophase values for pineal NYP are higher than those in photophase[22] and intra-arterial injection of NPY doubles pineal NAT activity,[23] NPY may potentiate pineal gland melatonin secretion.[24]

Opioid Peptides

Opioid peptides belong to several families of compounds with morphine-like pharmacological properties. One of these, β-endorphin is derived from proopiomelanocortin, the precursor of α-melanocyte-stimulating hormone (MSH) and

TABLE 1
Pineal Neuropeptides

Neuropeptide	Researchers[a]
Calcitonin gene-related peptide	Shiotani et al., 1986; Ruess et al., 1992
Delta sleep-inducting peptide	Graf et al., 1981; Graf and Kasting, 1986; Noteborn et al., 1988; Ouichou et al., 1992
Enkephalins	Schröder et al., 1988; Moore and Sibony, 1988; Møller et al., 1991; Aloyo, 1991; Coto-Montes et al., 1994
Luteinizing hormone-releasing hormone	Kastin et al., 1976; King and Millar, 1981; Matsuma and Sano, 1983
α-Melanocyte stimulating hormone	Sakai et al., 1976; Oliver and Porter, 1978; Vaudry et al., 1978; Pévet et al., 1980; O'Donohue et al., 1980; Trentini et al., 1980; Oaknin et al., 1986, 1987; Schröder et al., 1988
Natriuretic peptides	Olcese et al., 1994
Neuropeptide Y	Schon et al., 1985; Schröder, 1986; Schröder and Vollrath, 1986; Shiotani et al., 1986; Reuss and Schröder, 1987; Møller et al., 1988; Hexum et al., 1988; Williams et al., 1989; Møller et al., 1990; Mikkelsen and Møller, 1990; Olcese, 1991; Mikkelsen et al., 1991; Mikkelsen and Mick, 1992; Phansuwan-Pujito et al., 1993; Møller et al., 1994; Matsushima et al., 1994; Simmoneaux et al., 1994
Peptide histidine isoleucine	Møller and Mikkelsen, 1989
Pituitary-activating adenylate cyclase peptides	Masuo et al., 1992; Simonneaux et al., 1993; Yuwiler et al; 1995; Chik and Ho, 1995; Christophe, 1996; Schomerus et al., 1996
Secretoneurin	Simonneaux et al., 1997
Somatostatin	Pelletier et al., 1975; Findley et al., 1981; Webb and Peinad, 1986; Webb et al., 1984, 1989; Møller et al., 1992, 1994
Substance P	Rønnekleiv and Kelly, 1980, 1984; Korf and Møller, 1984; Shiotani et al., 1986, 1989; Rønnekleiv, 1988; Reuss et al., 1992; Møller et al., 1993; Matsushima et al., 1994
Vasointestinal peptide	Uddman et al., 1980; Møller et al., 1981, 1985; Møller and Korf, 1983; Korf and Møller, 1984; Møller and Mikkelsen, 1989; Shiotani et al., 1986; Mikkelsen et al., 1987; Cozzi et al, 1990, 1994; Møller et al., 1991; Piszczkiewicz and Zigmond, 1992
Vasopressin and oxytocin	Dogterom et al., 1978, 1980; Buijs and Pévet, 1980; Nurnberger and Korf, 1981; Matsura and Sano, 1983; Korf and Møller, 1984; Liu and Burback, 1987, 1988; Liu et al., 1987, 1991; Gauquelin et al., 1988; Rønnekleiv, 1988; Benson et al., 1990; Olcese et al., 1993; Lepetit et al., 1993; Matthews et al., 1993; Olcese et al., 1993

[a] For references to listed authors, refer to reviews by Ebadi et al.,[6] Pévet et al.,[9] Simonneaux,[10] Møller et al.,[12,13,49,56] Stankov et al.,[30] and Christophe.[36]

adrenocorticotropic hormone (ACTH). The others are derived from proenkephalin, which yields leucine-enkephalin (L-ENK) and methionine-enkephalin (M-ENK), and prodynorphin, the prohormone for dynorphins A and B. Most opioid peptides have been identified either in mammalian pineal nerve fibers or pinealocytes with considerable species differences in distribution reported (refer to Table 1). Moore and Sibony[25] demonstrated the presence of L-ENK in the human pineal gland in 1988. The origin of these and other opioidergic fibers is not known. Simonneaux[13] suggested on the basis of their distributions that opioid peptides present in pinealopetal fibers and/or pinealocytes may not only bring information from other parts of the body, but may serve a paracrine role, as well.

In vivo studies suggest a stimulatory role for opioid peptides on melatonin secretion.[26,27] Administration of the opioid receptor antagonist naloxone induced a decrease in nocturnal melatonin in rat pineals.[28] Conversely, endorphin, L-ENK, and M-ENK show no effects on melatonin release or pineal cAMP formation *in vitro*,[29,30] suggesting that these peptides do not act directly on pinealocyte membranes where delta opioid receptors have been identified.[31,32] An interesting relationship among opioid peptides, the pineal gland, and analgesia was suggested by Ebadi et al.[6]

Pituitary Activation Adenylate Cyclase Peptides

Pituitary activation adenylate cyclase peptides (PACAPs) were isolated from the hypothalamus by Miyata et al.[33] in 1989, and they are believed to play a variety of important physiological roles including a decrease in food intake and increases in arginine vasopressin and luteinizing hormone (LH) in rats.[34,35] PACAPs are members of the secretin/glucagon family of peptides which have been identified in the pineal gland (Table 1).

Pituitary activation adenylate cyclase peptide binding to rat pineal has been demonstrated,[36] and stimulation of melatonin secretion from the rat pineal gland was observed *in vitro* by Simonneaux et al.[37] High-affinity receptors have been identified for PACAP.[38,39] Recent reports suggest that PACAP increases NAT and melatonin content in rat pineals.[40,41] Chik and Ho[42] observed that PACAP increased pineal gland cAMP, but not cGMP, and potentiated α_1-adrenergic activation of melatonin secretion. Schomerus et al.[41] treated dispersed pinealocytes with varying concentrations of PACAP and analyzed effects on the cAMP response element binding protein. Compared to VIP, fewer pinealocytes responded to PACAP, and their response was more variable. In this study, it was suggested that both these neuropeptides are less effective than NE in stimulating melatonin synthesis.

Substance P

Substance P (SP) is a peptide of the tachykinin family. SP has been found in many areas of the nervous system, where it is thought to serve as a neurotransmitter in numerous physiological functions, including pituitary hormone release. SP-positive nerve fibers terminate in the perivascular spaces and between pinealocytes throughout the pineal gland but are probably not derived from the superior cervical ganglia.[43–46] Although high-affinity binding sites for SP have been identified in the bovine pineal gland,[47] no effect on melatonin secretion has been reported (see reviews by Simonneaux[13] and Møller et al.[48]).

Somatostatin

Somatostatin (SO), one of the first neuropeptides to be identified in the pineal gland, has a wide distribution in the central nervous system of mammalian species.[49] SO concentrations show nyctohemeral variations in rat pineals[50] and seasonal variations.[51] Despite these facts, studies on the effect of SO on melatonin secretion are equivocal.[13,21,30]

Vasoactive Intestinal Peptide and Histidine Isoleucine

Vasoactive intestinal peptide (VIP) and histidine isoleucine (PHI) are in the secretin/ glucagon family with PACAP, all three of which have been identified in the pineal gland. Interesting, superior cervical ganglionectomy does not modify VIP innervation in the pineal gland,[52–54] indicating that pineal VIP innervation may be of extrasympathetic origin and may derive from the pterygopalatine ganglia[45] or be of central origin.[11,55] VIP stimulates pineal cAMP, NAT, and melatonin secretion[13,30,37,53,56,57] and increases intracellular calcium.[58] VIP stimulation of melatonin synthesis potentiates concomitant activation of α_1-adrenergic receptors.[56,59] VIP was shown by Moujir et al.[60] to be without effects on NAT and melatonin synthesis in hamster pineals. Simonneaux[13] points out that while it is clear from several studies that VIP is a potent activator of melatonin synthesis, the information brought to the pineal by pinealopetal neurons containing this neuropeptide has not been determined. Because light increases VIP binding sites in the pineal and the cAMP response to VIP and pineal VIP shows nyctohemeral variations, Simonneaux suggests that VIP may be involved in the transmission of information about lighting conditions.

Vasopressin and Oxytocin

Vasopressin (VP)- and oxytocin (OT)-containing nerve fibers are derived from the habenular commissure and terminate frequently in pineal gland perivascular spaces. Thus, it is thought that they are of central origin. Many of these fibers may be derived from the paraventricular nuclei.[44] Although VP or OT have not been identified in pinealocyte perikaria, VP mRNA expression has been reported recently for several species.[61-63]

Controversy exists between several studies in which VP effects on melatonin were examined *in vivo* and *in vitro,* raising questions about binding sites and species variations in response. Simonneaux et al.[13,18,64] suggest that VP potentiates the NE-induced activation of melatonin synthesis via specific receptors.

Although pineal concentrations of OT show temporal variations, increasing with VP at night,[65,66] the relationship to nocturnal increases in melatonin synthesis has not been established, and the effects of OT have not been extensively explored.

Secretoneurin and Other Neuropeptides

Secretoneurin (SN) is a 33-amino-acid peptide found in the central and sympathetic nervous system. Simonneaux et al.[67] recently investigated the presence of SN in the rat pineal gland and its effect on serotonin and melatonin release. This novel neuropeptide was discovered in higher amounts in the hamster than in the rat gland. SN was observed in nerve fibers in the parenchyma and pineal stalk in rats, but was not localized to rat pinealocytes. SN was seen, however, in a population of hamster pinealocytes. In culture with rat pinealocytes, SN demonstrated significant inhibitory effects on serotonin and melatonin release.

Other neuropeptides include calcitonin gene-related peptide (CGRP) observed in rat and gerbil pineal[45,46] and natriuretic peptides. The latter have been shown to activate specific pinealocyte receptors and increase cGMP without significant effects on melatonin secretion.[22]

It has been known for many years that the neuropeptide gonadotropin releasing hormone (GnRH) is present in sheep pineals, in which concentrations demonstrate seasonal changes.[68] GnRH (LHRH) was identified in cells located in the habenular and commissural areas that project to the pineal gland in the dog,[69] and Mess et al. showed in 1991[21] that GnRH stimulates melatonin release from perifused rat pineal glands. More recently, Benson and Ebels[70] isolated a decapeptide from bovine pineal gland extracts that demonstrates antigonadotropic effects.

Classification of Pineal Neuropeptides

The diverse neuropeptides identified in the pineal gland have been classified by Pévet[8,71] based on whether or not they are (1) taken up from the circulation, (2) are present in pinealopetal nerves and serve as modulators of adrenergic-stimulated melatonin synthesis, or (3) are pineal peptides synthesized and secreted by pinealocytes. These classifications are illustrated in Figure 1.

Since the pineal gland is outside the blood brain barrier and its capillaries are fenestrated, some investigators have assumed that many peptides are taken up by the pineal from the circulation quite readily (category 1, above). On the contrary, however,

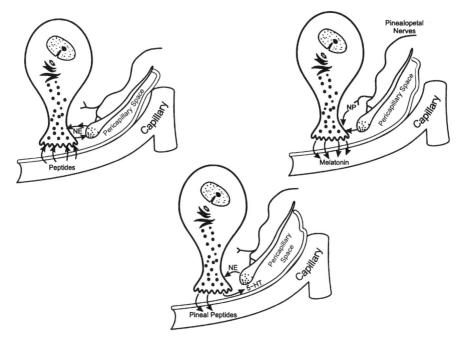

FIGURE 1

Classification of pineal neuropeptides. Upper left demonstrates peptides leaving the circulation, crossing a thin basal lamina, and being taken up by a pinealocyte polar process. A norepinephrine (NE)-containing nerve ending is seen in the pericapillary space. Modulation of melatonin secretion by a neuropeptide (NP)-containing pinealopetal nerve is shown in the upper right. In the lower center, a pinealocyte is depicted releasing neuropeptide secretory product in association with serotonin (5-HT).

only a few have actually been shown to be taken up from pineal gland circulation. These include LHRH,[72] α-melanocyte-stimulating hormone,[73,74] and delta sleep-inducing peptide (DSIP).[75–77]

Peptides known to be synthesized by the pineal (category 3) are equally few. To date, pineal synthesis has been demonstrated only for enkephalins,[78,79] vasopressin,[61–63] and somatostatin by Møller et al. (see footnote in Reference 8). And, while a number of neuropeptides may serve as modulators of melatonin secretion (category 2), as reviewed above, many others identified in the pineal gland have not been adequately related to a known pineal function and probably serve some function that remains unidentified.

Summary

While it is well established that sympathetic post-ganglionic fibers innervate the mammalian pineal gland and stimulate melatonin synthesis, evidence has accumulated in recent years that other neurotransmitters and neuropeptides are present in the pineal gland that potentially play a role in the regulation of indoleamine synthesis. While the stimulatory or inhibitory effects on melatonin secretion of a number of neuropeptides have been examined, the role of most neuropeptides localized to the pineal gland have not been studied extensively. Several that have been examined demonstrate no effect *in vitro,* and the effects of others were found to be equivocal. VP is an example of a neuropeptide that falls into the latter group. Neuropeptides shown to have the potential to increase melatonin secretion include LHRH, DSIP, VIP, PACAP, and OP. On the other hand, NPY and SN, a novel neuropeptide studied recently by Simonneaux et al.,[70] demonstrate significant inhibitory effects on melatonin synthesis and secretion.

References

1. Moore, R.Y., The innervation of the mammalian pineal gland, in Reiter, R.J., Ed., *Progress in Reproductive Biology.* Vol. 4. *The Pineal and Reproduction,* S. Karger, New York, 1978, 1.

2. Brooks, C., Ishikawa, M.C., and Koizumi, A., Autonomic system control of the pineal gland and the role of this complex in the integration of body function, *Brain Res.,* 87, 181, 1975.

3. Ariens Kappers, J., The development, topographical relations and innervation of the epiphysis cerebri in the albino rat, *Z. Zellforsch.,* 52, 163. 1960.

4. Klein, D.C., Sugden, D., and Weller, J.C., Postsynaptic α-adrenergic receptors potentiate the β-adrenergic stimulation of pineal serotonin-*N*-acetyl transferase, *Proc. Natl. Acad. Sci. USA,* 80, 599, 1983.

5. Ebadi, M. and Govitrapong, P., Orphan transmitters and their receptor sites in the pineal gland, in Reiter, R.J., Ed., *Pineal Research Reviews,* Vol 4, Alan R. Liss, New York, 1986, 1.

6. Ebadi, M., Hexum, T.D., Pfeiffer, R.F., and Govitrapong, P., Pineal and retinal peptides and their receptors, in Reiter, R.J., Ed., *Pineal Research Reviews,* Vol. 7, Alan R. Liss, New York, 1989, 1.

7. Vivien-Röels, B., Masson-Pévet, M., Canguilhem, B., Bonn, D., and Pévet, P., Effect of photoperiod on the daily rhythm of pineal and/or circulating melatonin and 5-methoxytryptophol (ML) concentrations in the European hamster, *Cricetus cricetus,* in Touitou, Y., Arendt, J., and Pévet, P., Eds., *Melatonin and the Pineal Gland — From Basic Science to Clinical Application,* Elsevier, Amsterdam, 1993, 199.

8. Pévet, P., Physiological role of neuropeptides in the mammalian pineal gland, in Foldes, A. and Reiter, R.J., Eds., *Advances in Pineal Research,* Vol. 6, John Libbey & Co., London, 1991, 275.

9. Coto-Montes, A., Masson-Pévet, M., Pévet, P., and Møller, M., The presence of opioidergic pinealocytes in the pineal gland of the European hamster (*Cricetus cricetus*): an immunocytochemical study, *Cell Tiss. Res.,* 278, 483, 1994.

10. Møller, M., Cozzi, M., Schröder, H., and Mikkelsen, J.D., The peptidergic innervation of the mammalian pineal gland, in Trentini, G.P., DeGaetini, C., and Pévet, P., Eds., *Fundamentals and Clinics in Pineal Research*, Raven Press, New York, 1987, 71.

11. Møller, M., The fine structure of the pinealopetal innervation of the mammalian pineal gland, *J. Microsc. Res. Technol.*, 21, 188, 1992.

12. Møller, M., Ravault, J.P., and Cozzi, B., The neuroanatomy of the mammalian pineal gland: neuropeptides, *Neurochem. Int.*, 28, 23, 1996.

13. Simonneaux, V., Neuropeptides of the mammalian pineal gland, *Neuroendocrinol. Lett.*, 17, 115, 1995.

14. Card, J.P. and Moore, R.Y., Organization of lateral geniculate-hypothalamic connections in the rat, *J. Comp. Neurol.*, 284, 135, 1989.

15. Mikkelsen, J.D. and Møller, M., A direct neural projection from the intergeniculate leaflet of the lateral geniculate nucleus to the deep pineal gland of the rat, demonstrated with *Phaseolus vulgaris* leucoaggutinin, *Brain Res.*, 520, 342, 1990.

16. Mikkelsen, J.D., Cozzi, B., and Møller, M., Efferent projections from the lateral geniculate nucleus to the pineal complex of the Mongolian gerbil (*Meriones unguiculatus*), *Cell Tissue Res.*, 264, 95, 1991.

17. Vacas, M.I., Keller-Sarmiento, M.I., Pereyra, E.N., Etchegoyen, G.S., and Cardinali D.P., *In vitro* effect of neuropeptide Y on melatonin and norepinephrine release in rat pineal gland, *Cell Mol. Neurobiol.*, 7, 309, 1987.

18. Simonneaux, V., Ouichou, A., Craft, C., and Pévet, P., Presynaptic and postsynaptic effects of neuropeptide Y in the rat pineal gland, *J. Neurochem.*, 62, 2464, 1994.

19. Olcese, J., Neuropeptide Y: an endogenous inhibitor of norepinephrine-stimulated melatonin secretion in the rat pineal gland, *J. Neurochem.*, 57, 943, 1991.

20. Harada, Y., Okubo, M., Yaga, K., Kaneko, T., and Kaku, K., Neuropeptide Y inhibits β-adrenergic agonist- and vasoactive intestinal peptide-induced cyclic AMP accumulation in rat pinealocytes through pertussis toxin-sensitive G protein, *J. Neurochem.*, 59, 2178, 1992.

21. Arendt, J., *Melatonin and the Mammalian Pineal Gland*, Chapman and Hall, London, 1995, 60.

22. Olcese, J., Muller, D., Munker, M., and Schmidt, C., Natriuretic peptides elevate cyclic 3′,5′-guanosine monophosphate levels in cultured rat pinealocytes: evidence for guanylate cyclase-linked membrane receptors, *Mol. Cell. Endocrinol.*, 103, 95, 1994.

23. Reuss, S. and Schröder, H., Neuropeptide Y effects on pineal melatonin synthesis in the rat, *Neurosci. Lett.*, 74, 128, 1987.

24. Alberts, H.E. and Ferris, C.F., Neuropeptide Y role in light-dark cycle entrainment of hamster circadian rhythms, *Neurosci. Lett.*, 50, 163, 1984.

25. Moore, R.Y. and Siboni, P., Enkephalin-like immunoreactivity in neurons in the human pineal gland, *Brain Res.*, 457, 395, 1988.

26. Fraschini, F., Esposti, D., Esposti, G., Lucini, V., Mariani, M., Scaglione, F., Vignati, G., and Dela Bella, D., On a possible role of endogenous opioid peptides on melatonin secretion, in Reiter, R.J. and Pang, S.F., Eds., *Advances in Pineal Research*, Vol. 3, Libbey, London, 1989, 61.

27. Gaffori, O.M. and van Ree, J.M., Des-tyr[1]-γ-endorphin and haloperidol increase pineal gland melatonin levels in rats, *Peptides,* 4, 393, 1983.

28. Lowenstein, P.R., Pereyra, E.N., Solveyra, C.G., and Cardinali, D.P., Effect of naloxone on the nocturnal rise of rat pineal melatonin content, *Eur. J. Pharmacol.,* 98, 261, 1984.

29. Stankov, B., Esposti, D., Esposti, K.G., Lucini, V., Mariani, M., Cozzi, K.B., Scaglione, F., and Fraschini, F., Opioid involvement in the control of melatonin synthesis and release, in Reiter, R.J. and Lukaszyk, A., Eds., *Advances in Pineal Research,* Vol. 4, Libbey, London, 1990, 45.

30. Kaneko, T., Cheng, P.Y., Oka, H., Oda, T., Yanaihara, N., and Yanaihara, C., Vasoactive intestinal polypeptide stimulates adenylate cyclase and serotonin *N*-acetyl transferase activities in rat pineal *in vitro, Biomed. Res.,* 1, 84, 1980.

31. Aloyo, V.J., Identification and characterization of delta opioid binding sites in the bovine pineal, *J. Pharmacol. Exp. Ther.,* 262, 292, 1992.

32. Govitrapong, P., Pariyanonth, M., and Ebadi, M., The presence and actions of opioid receptors in bovine pineal gland, *J. Pineal Res.,* 13, 124, 1992.

33. Miyata, A., Arimura, A., Dah., R.R., Minamino, N., Uehara, A., Jiang, L., Culler, M.D., and Coy, D.H., Isolation of a novel 38 residue-hypothalamic polypeptide which stimulates adenylate cyclase in pituitary cells, *Biochem. Biophys. Res. Comm.,* 164, 567, 1989.

34. Arimura, A. and Shioda, S., Pituitary adenylate cyclase activating polypeptide (PACAP) and its receptors: neuroendocrine and endocrine interaction, *Frontiers Neuroendocrinol.,* 16, 53, 1995.

35. Christophe, J., Type I receptors for PACAP (a neuropeptide even more important than VIP?), *Biochim. Biophys. Acta,* 1154, 183, 1993.

36. Masuo, Y., Ohtaki, T., Masuda, Y., Tsuda, M., and Fujino, M., Binding sites for pituitary and adenylate cyclase activating polypeptide (PACAP): comparison with vasoactive intestinal polypeptide (VIP) binding site localization in rat brain sections, *Brain Res.,* 575, 113, 1992.

37. Simonneax, V., Ouichou, A., and Pévet, P., Pituitary adenylate cyclase-activating polypeptide (PACAP) stimulates melatonin synthesis from rat pineal gland, *Brain Res.,* 603, 148, 1993.

38. Olcese, J., McArdle, C., Mikkelsen, J.D., and Hannibal, J., PACAP and type I PACAP receptors in the pineal gland, *Ann. N.Y. Acad. Sci.,* 805, 595, 1996.

39. Nelsson, S.F., DeNeef, P., Robberecht, P., and Christophe, J., Characterization of ocular receptors for PACAP and their coupling to adenylate cyclase, *Exp. Eye Res.,* 58, 459, 1994.

40. Yuwiler, A., Brammer, G.L., and Bennett, B.L., Interaction between adrenergic and peptide stimulation in the rat pineal: pituitary adenylate cyclase-activating peptide, *J. Neurochem.,* 64, 2273, 1995.

41. Schomerus, C.S., Maronde, E., Laedtke, E., and Korf, H.-W., Vasoactive intestinal peptide (VIP) and pituitary adenylate cyclase-activating polypeptide (PACAP) induce phosphorylation of the transcription factor CREB in subpopulations of rat pinealocytes: immunocytochemical and immunochemical evidence, *Cell Tissue Res.,* 286, 305, 1996.

42.   Chik, C.L. and Ho, A.K., Pituitary adenylate cyclase-activating polypeptide: control of rat pineal cyclic AMP and melatonin but not GMP, *J. Neurochem.*, 64, 2111, 1995.

43.   Rønnekleiv, O.K. and Kelly, M.J., Distribution of substance P neurons in the epithalamus of the rat: an immunohistochemical investigation, *J. Pineal Res.*, 1, 355, 1984.

44.   Korf, H.-W. and Møller, M., The innervation of the mammalian pineal gland with special references to central pinealopetal projections, in Reiter, R.J., Ed., *Pineal Research Reviews*, Vol. 2, Alan R. Liss, New York, 1984, p. 41.

45.   Shiotani, Y., Yamono, M., Shiosaka, S., Emson, P.C., Hillyard, C.J., Girgis, S., and MacIntyre, I., Distribution and origins of substance P (SP)-, calcitonin gene-related peptide (CGRP)-, vasoactive intestinal polypeptide (VIP)-, and neuropeptide Y (NPY)-containing nerve fibers in the pineal gland of gerbils, *Neurosci. Lett.*, 70, 187, 1986.

46.   Reuss, S., Riemann, R., and Vollrath, L., Substance P- and calcitonin gene related peptide-like immunoreactive neurons in the rat trigeminal ganglion — with special reference to meningeal and pineal innervation, *Acta Histochem.*, 92, 104, 1992.

47.   Govitrapong, P. and Ebadi, M., Studies on high-affinity [^{3}H] substance P binding sites in bovine pineal gland, *Endocrinol. Res.*, 12, 293, 1986.

48.   Møller, M., Ravault, J.P., and Cozzi, B., The neuroanatomy of the mammaian pineal gland: neuropeptides, *Neurochem. Int.*, 28, 23, 1996.

49.   Pelletier, G., Leclerc, R., Dube, D., Labrie, F., Puviane, R., Arimura, A., and Schally, A.V., Localization of growth hormone-release-inhibiting hormone (somatostatin) in the rat brain, *Am. J. Anat.*, 141, 397, 1975.

50.   Møller, M., Mikkelsen, J.D., Holst, J.J., and Phansuwan-Pujiton, P., Somatostatin and prosomatostatin immunoreactive nerve fibers in the bovine pineal gland, *Neuroendocrinology*, 56, 278, 1992.

51.   Webb, S.M., Champney, T.H., Steger, R.W., Bartke, A., and Reiter, R.J., Immunoreactive somatostatin in the pineal gland of different rodent species: circadian rhythm, effect of superior cervical ganglionectomy, pineal indole administration and lighting conditions, *Biomed. Res.*, 5, 473, 1984.

52.   Morgan, P.J., Williams, L.M., Lawson, W., and Riddoch, G., Adrenergic and VIP stimulation of cyclic AMP accumulation in ovine pineals, *Brain Res.*, 447, 279, 1988.

53.   Yuweiler, A., Vasoactive intestinal peptide stimulation of pineal serotonin-N-acetyltransferase activity: general characteristics, *J. Neurochem.*, 41, 146, 1983.

54.   Piszczkiewicz, S. and Zigmond, R.E., Is the vasoactive intestinal peptide-like immunoreactivity in the rat pineal gland present in fibers originating in the superior cervical ganglion?, *Brain Res.*, 589, 327, 1992.

55.   Cozzi, B., Mikkelsen, J.D., Ravault, R.-P., Locatelli, A., Fahrenkrug, J., Zhang, E.-T., and Møller, M., Density of peptide histidine-, isoleucine-, and vasoactive intestinal peptide-immunoreactive nerve fibers in the sheep pineal gland is not affected by superior cervical ganglionectomy, *J. Comp. Neurol.*, 343, 72, 1994.

56.   Ho, A.K., Chik, C.L., and Klein, D.C., Transmembrane receptor cross-talk: concurrent VIP and alpha-1-adrenergic activation rapidly elevates pinealocyte cGMP greater than 100-fold, *Biochem. Biophys. Res. Comm.*, 146, 1478, 1987.

57. Simonneaux, V., Ouichou, A., and Pévet, P., Vasoactive intestinal peptide stimulates melatonin release from perifused pineal glands of rats, *J. Neural Trans.*, 79, 69, 1990.

58. Shaad, N.C., Vanecek, J., Rodriquez, I.R., Klein, D.C., Holtzclaw, L., Russel, J.T., Vasoactive intestinal peptide elevates pinealocyte intracellular calcium concentrations by enhancing influx: evidence for involvement of a cyclic GMP-dependent mechanism, *Mol. Pharmacol.*, 47, 923, 1995.

59. Yuweiler, A., Synergistic action of postsynaptic α-adrenergic receptor stimulation on vasoactive intestinal polypeptide-induced increases in pineal *N*-acetyltransferase, *J. Neurochem.*, 49, 806, 1987.

60. Moujir, F., Richardson, B.A., Yaga, K., and Reiter, R.J., Vasoactive intestinal peptide stimulates *N*-acetyltransferase and hydroxyindole-*O*-methyltransferase activities and melatonin production in cultured rat but not in Syrian hamster pineal glands, *J. Pineal Res.*, 12, 35, 1992.

61. Lepetit, P., Fever-Montange, M., Gay, N., Belin, M.-F., and Bobillier, P., Vasopressin mRNA in the cerebellum and circumventricular organs: a quantitative *in situ* hybridization study, *Neurosci. Lett.*, 159, 171, 1993.

62. Matthews, S.G., Parrott, R.F., and Sirinathsinghji, D.J.S., Distribution and cellular localization of vasopressin mRNA in the ovine brain, pituitary and pineal glands, *Neuropeptides*, 25, 11, 1993.

63. Olcese, J., Sinemus, C., and Ivell, R., Vasopressin innervation of the bovine pineal gland: is there a local source for arginine vasopressin?, *Mol. Cell. Neurosci.*, 4, 47, 1993.

64. Simonneax, V., Ouichou, A., Burbach, J.P.H., and Pévet, P., Vasopressin and oxytocin modulation of melatonin secretion from rat pineal glands, *Peptides*, 11, 1075, 1990.

65. Liu, B. and Burbach, J.P.H., Circadian variations of vasopressin level and vasopressin-converting amino peptidase activity in the rat pineal gland, *Peptides*, 9, 973, 1988.

66. Gauquelin, G., Gharib, C., Ghaemmaghami, F., Allevard, A.-M., Cherbal, F., Geelen, G., Bouzeghrane, F., and Legros, J.-J., A day/night rhythm of vasopressin and oxytocin in rat retina, pineal and harderian gland, *Peptides*, 9, 289, 1988.

67. Simonneaux, V., Vuillez, P., Eder, U., Miguez, J.M., Pévet, P., and Fischer-Colbrie, R., Secretoneurin: a new neuropeptide in the rodent pineal gland, *Cell Tiss. Res.*, 288, 427, 1997.

68. King, J.A. and Millar, R.P., Decapeptide luteinizing hormone-releasing hormone in ovine pineal gland, *J. Endocrinol.*, 91, 405, 1981.

69. Matsuura, T. and Sano, Y., Distribution of monoamine-containing nerve fibers in the pineal organ of untreated and sympathectomized dogs, *Cell Tissue Res.*, 234, 519, 1983.

70. Benson, B. and Ebels, I., Structure of a pineal gland-derived antigonadotropic decapeptide, *Life Sci.*, 54, PL437, 1994.

71. Pévet, P., The different classes of proteic and peptidic substances present in the pineal gland, in Axelrod, J., Fraschini, F., and Velo, G.P., Eds., *The Pineal Gland and Its Endocrine Role*, Plenum Press, New York, 1983, 113.

72. Kastin, A.J., Nissen, C., Nikolics, K., Medzihradszky, K., Coy, D.P., Teplan, I., and Schally, A.V., Distribution of ³H-alpha-MSH in rat brain, *Brain Res. Bull.,* 1, 19, 1976.

73. Sakai, K.K., Schneider, D., Felt, F., and Marks, B.H., The effect of α-MSH on β-adrenergic receptor mechanisms in the rat pineal, *Life Sci.,* 19, 1145, 1976.

74. Trentini, G.P., DeGaetini, C.F., DiGregorio, C., and Boticelli, C.S., LHRH incorporation in normal and denervated pineal gland, and in pineal glands of rats with constant estrous-anovulatory syndrome: a preliminary study, *Endocrinologie,* 76, 6, 1980.

75. Graf, M.V., Lorez, H.P., Gillessen, D., Tobler, H.J., and Schoenberger, G.A., Distribution and specific binding of ³H-labeled DSIP, *Experientia,* 37, 625, 1981.

76. Graf, M.V. and Kastin, A.J., Delta sleep inducing peptide (DSIP): an update, *Peptides,* 7, 1165, 1986.

77. Ouichou, A., Zitouni, M., Raynaud, F., Simonneaux, V., Gharib, A., and Pévet, P., Delta-sleep-inducing peptide stimulates melatonin, 5-methoxytryptophol and serotonin secretion from perifused rat pineal glands, *Biol. Signals,* 1, 65, 1992.

78. Aloyo, V.J., Preproenkephalin A gene expression in rat pineal, *Neuroendocrinology,* 54, 594, 1991.

79. Coto-Montes, A., Masson-Pévet, M., Pévet, P., and Møller, M., The presence of opioidergic pinealocytes in the pineal gland of the European hamster (*Cricetus cricetus*): an immunocytochemical study, *Cell Tissue Res.,* 278, 483, 1994.

Chapter 9

Pineal Gland-Derived Antigonadotropic Decapeptide

Bryant Benson

Contents

Introduction

Although microscopic studies on mammalian pineal glands clearly demonstrate morphological characteristics consistent with cells that synthesize a protein secretory product,[1,2] the search for unique antigonadotropic peptides synthesized and secreted by pinealocytes has a long and arduous history. Numerous individuals and groups have worked on this problem since the 1930s, and, in general, their results have yielded more questions than answers.[3–8]

0-8493-8564-4/99/$0.00+$.50

Mammalian pinealocytes contain rough endoplasmic reticulum and elaborate Golgi complexes often with associated secretory vesicles which migrate along elongated cytoplasmic processes oriented in their projection toward pineal capillaries. Clear secretory vesicles or dense-cored granules containing protein material are apparently released from pinealocyte polar terminals in peripapillary spaces. Such secretory products have ready access to the blood, as generally they have only to traverse a thin basal lamina and capillaries that are, for the most part, fenestrated. Melatonin has not been localized to pinealocyte secretory vesicles or dense-cored granules, whereas serotonin has in association with an unidentified secretory protein.[9,10] The probability that secretory vesicles contain a major, unidentified protein secretory product in association with serotonin places pinealocytes in the "APUD" category of cells,[11] a series of endocrine cells that share the property of production and secretion of polypeptide hormones. Such cells are capable of amine precursor uptake (APU) and contain amino acid decarboxylase (D) and a high content of nonspecific esterase or cholinesterase. Pinealocytes fulfill these conditions, confirming that they are indeed endocrine cells, or paraneurons,[12,13] even though the chemical nature of the protein secretory product remains undetermined.

Some 10 years ago, we completed a computer-enhanced comparative study of rat brain region peptides and proteins, including the pineal gland.[14] The methods included two-dimensional polyacrylamide gel electrophoresis, silver staining, and computer analysis. In this study, protein spot mapping and characterizations of molecular weight and isoelectric points (pI) were compiled and comparisons made between acidic extracts of the pineal gland, retina, hypothalamus, and cerebral cortex. This extensive study identified 17 proteins unique to the pineal gland and several others common to the retina and pineal gland that were not found in cerebral cortex. The function of these unique pineal proteins is unknown, but no doubt some relate to indoleamine synthesis and others may function in the synthesis of neuropeptide secretory products which remain unidentified.

Search for Antigonadotropic Peptides

Over the years, we observed antigonadotropic effects of partially purified peptidic extracts of rat, human, bovine, and ovine glands after injection in rodents. The effects in rats and mice included reduction of gonad and accessory weights, blockage of compensatory ovarian hypertrophy, inhibition of post-castration rises in luteinizing hormone (LH) and follicle-stimulating hormone (FSH), reduction of prolactin (PRL) and LH in intact animals, delay of puberty, reduction of fertility, and blockage of ovulation.[3,4,8,15,16] In most of these studies, peptides were extracted from defatted bovine or ovine pineal glands with dilute acetic acid, and, after serial ultrafiltration through Amicon ultrafiltration membranes, small molecular weight peptides were separated by Sephadex chromatography. When ion exchange chromatography was applied,[17] we learned early on that the peptides with antigonadotropic properties shared chromatographic properties with oxytocin (OT), and not with vasopressin (VP) or the putative pineal antigonadotropin arginine vasotocin (AVT).

Eventually, a large-scale extraction was completed with the aim of determining the structure of peptides with demonstrated neurohypophysial-like activity (mouse mammary milk-ejection assay) and those with antigonadotropic (anti-LH/anti-PRL) activity. These studies utilized 10 kg of bovine pineal glands (approximately 250,000 glands) and took 6 years to complete.[18,19] After final purification by serial preparative high-performance liquid chromatography, primary structures were determined by automated amino acid and microsequence analyses. The study concluded that the peptides responsible for neurohypophysial hormone-like activity were VP and OT. AVT was not identified in bovine pineals. The structure of a novel antigonadotropic decapeptide (AGD) was revealed. Purified AGD, as well as synthetic analogs, were seen to reduce circulating levels of PRL and LH after acute intra-arterial or intra-atrial injection in male rats.

Effects of AGD on PRL

Other experiments were performed to determine whether chronic lateral ventricle infusion of AGD would depress circulating PRL levels in conscious, freely moving male rats. Artificial cerebrospinal fluid (CSF) at a rate of 1.0 µl/hr, or the AGD in CSF (0.5 µg/1.0 µl/hr) were infused over a period of 7 days into the right lateral ventricles via subcutaneous Alzet osmotic mini-pumps attached to stereotaxically fitted intra-cerebroventricular cannulae. As in previous experiments, indwelling intra-arterial Tygon microbore cannulae permitted the morning and late afternoon sampling of blood for the determination of PRL concentrations by radioimmunoassay. Circulating PRL concentrations were significantly depressed by AGD infusion, both in the morning and late afternoon on infusion days 4 through 7. At sacrifice after 7 days of AGD infusion, it was noted that pituitary concentrations of PRL were significantly increased concomitant with decreased serum PRL levels.[20]

Effects of Acute Intra-Arterial Injection of AGD on Stress-Induced PRL Release

A recent report suggested that AGD attenuates stress-related increases in PRL secretion.[21] Additional experiments have confirmed these preliminary results. In the first experiment, ten young adult SD male rats were fitted with intra-arterial microbore cannulae for blood collection. On the morning of the next day, initial blood samples were drawn for PRL determination by radioimmunoassay. Following the retrieval of this blood sample, each was given either an intra-arterial injection of 0.2 ml saline or a bolus injection of 25 µg of the AGD in 0.2 ml of saline (time 0), and immediately exposed to diethyl ether for 2 min before blood samples were drawn at 5, 15, and 30 min. Although the ether stress-induced increase in PRL was not altered by AGD treatment at 5 minutes (Figure 1), AGD treatment significantly reduced PRL levels at 15 ($p < 0.01$) and 30 minutes ($p < 0.05$).

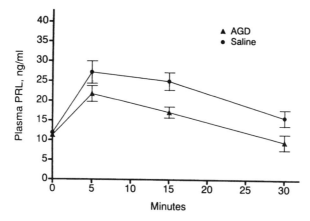

FIGURE 1

Effects of AGD on ether stress-induced PRL release. An intra-arterial injection of 25 μg of a synthetic analog of AGD depressed serum PRL levels at 15 and 30 min after a 2-min exposure of male rats to dimethyl ether.

The results of the first experiment were not unexpected, as in previous experiments in which AGD has been given to non-stressed rats by acute intra-arterial injection, maximum effects on PRL were observed at 30 min post-injection. Consequently, in a second experiment, male rats fitted with intra-arterial cannulae were given 25 μg of the AGD 25 min prior to ether exposure (for 2 min) which began at time 0. Blood samples were taken for PRL determination at 3 min prior to ether exposure, and at 5, 15, and 30 min afterwards. As shown in Figure 2, PRL levels in AGD-treated rats were significantly reduced ($p < 0.01$) 3 min prior to ether exposure (or 22 min after AGD injection), and the stress response to ether exposure significantly attenuated ($p < 0.01$) at 5 min after ether (or 30 min post-AGD injection).

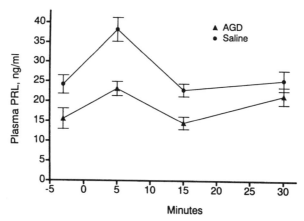

FIGURE 2

Effects of prior treatment with AGD on ether stress-induced PRL release. When given by bolus intra-arterial injection 25 min before exposure to dimethyl ether, 25 μg of AGD significantly reduced the PRL stress response at 5 and 15 min.

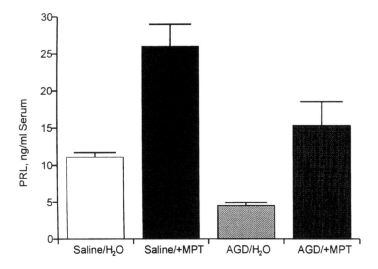

FIGURE 3
Effects of α-methyl-*p*-paratyrosine (MPT) on serum PRL levels in saline- or AGD-treated male rats. The increase in serum PRL levels seen after MPT treatment was significantly reduced in AGD-treated rats compared with saline-treated controls.

Effects of AGD on Hypothalamic Dopamine Turnover

Sixty-five young adult male SD rats were acclimatized for a period of 3 weeks to conditions of controlled photoperiod (L12:D12, lights on at 06.00 hr) and ambient temperature (22°C). On the morning of the experiment, 24 rats were given 50 μg of AGD by intra-atrial injection, and 24 others saline, 30 min prior to treatment with α-methyl-*p*-tyrosine (α-MPT) at time 0. For estimates of turnover rates, groups of eight AGD- or saline diluent-treated rats were killed at 30, 60, and 90 min after the intraperitoneal injection of α-MPT (250 mg/kg). For measurements of steady-state catecholamine concentrations ($[CA]_o$), additional groups of rats were given saline and killed at 0, 30, 60, and 90 min post-injection. Monoamine concentrations were determined in rapidly dissected medial basal hypothalamic/median eminence (MBH/ME) blocks by a method established in our laboratory.[22] Rate constants (k) for NE and DA disappearance were calculated by the method of least squares after log transformation. Estimates of synthesis (K), or turnover rates, were calculated using the formula $K = k[CA]_o$. Significant differences were determined by analysis of variance followed by the Newman-Keuls multiple range test.

As shown in Figure 3, the increase in circulating PRL levels after α-MPT treatment was diminished in AGD-treated rats compared with saline-treated controls. Also, the rate of MBH/ME DA depletion after α-MPT injection was significantly greater in AGD-treated rats compared with salient diluent-treated controls (Figure 4). Although higher, mean steady-state DA concentrations ($[DA]_o$) in the MBH/ME of

AGD-treated rats (1.42 ± 0.11 ng/mg protein) were not significantly different from control values at time 0 (1.38 ± 0.09 ng/mg protein). Conversely, the rate constant k (hr^{-1}) for DA depletion was significantly higher for AGD-treated rats (0.793 ± 0.087 ng/mg protein per hr) after α-MPT compared with that for diluent-treated controls (0.533 ± 0.043 ng/mg protein per hr; $p < 0.01$) as was the turnover rate, K. K for control rats was 0.735 ± 0.062 vs. 1.126 ± 0.093 ng/mg protein per hr for AGD-treated rats ($p < 0.01$). K for norepinephrine (data not shown) was not significantly different between control and AGD-treated rats.

Lack of an Effect of AGD on PRL Release *In Vitro*

In an attempt to determine whether AGD inhibited pituitary PRL secretion directly, female rat pituitaries were dispersed in cell culture with PRL levels measured *in vitro*. More than ten experiments were carried out with a variety of AGD concentrations (10^{-3} to 10^{-6} M) and diverse sample collection times. In no experiment was attenuation or inhibition of PRL release into the incubation medium observed. A sample experiment is shown in Figure 5, in which the concentration of AGD added to the medium is 1.0×10^{-5} M.

Effects of AGD on LH

While the depressive effects of AGD on PRL have been observed consistently, inhibitory effects of acute treatment on LH yielded inconsistent results after intravenous, intra-atrial, or intra-arterial injection in rats. On the other hand, infusion of small amounts of synthetic AGD into the lateral cerebral ventricles of castrated male rats significantly depressed LH pulse frequency and nadirs.[8,23] Because changing patterns of LH pulse frequency and amplitude are known to serve a physiological purpose in seasonal breeders where variability in these parameters plays a crucial role in switching gonadal function on and off,[24] studies were initiated in which the AGD is currently being tested in ewes at different times of year. Preliminary results indicate that intraventricular infusion of AGD modifies, and in some cases inhibits altogether, pulsatile LH release.[25,26]

Localization of AGD mRNA by Northern Hybridization

Standard northern analysis was performed to identify mRNA expression for AGD in rat tissues (Figure 6). Aliquots of mRNA extracted from rat pineals, hypothalami, and other tissues were subjected to electrophoresis on 1.0% agarose gels. The separated mRNA was transferred by positive pressure blotting onto Zeta-probe nylon

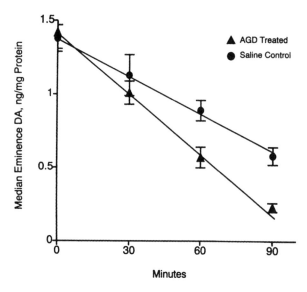

FIGURE 4
Increased turnover of dopamine (DA) in hypothalamic median eminence strips from rats treated with a
single, intra-arterial injection of AGD.

membranes and cross-linked to the membrane by exposure to ultraviolet radiation.
M_r markers were included on each gel and visualized under ultraviolet illumination
following staining with ethidium bromide. An anti-sense AGD oligonucleotide probe
was utilized (5' to 3' sequence = GGG GAA GTA GGT TTT GGT GGT GGG GAA
GGA). The probe was labeled at the 3' end with ^{32}P-dATP before pre-hybridization

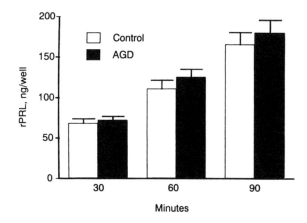

FIGURE 5
Lack of an effect of AGD on PRL release *in vitro*. Anterior pituitaries from female SD rats were incubated
in Dulbecco's modified Eagle's medium in the presence or absence of AGD (10^{-5} M). PRL release was
not affected by AGD treatment.

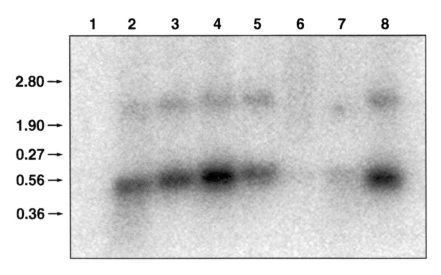

FIGURE 6

Northern analysis with an oligonucleotide AGD probe yielded hybridization bands between rat (lane 4) and steer (lane 8) pineals. Molecular weight markers were spotted in lane 1, as indicated on the left side of the illustration. Lane 2 = rat anterior hypothalamus; lane 3 = hypothalamic median eminence; lane 5 = rat corpus striatum; lane 6 = rat cerebellum; lane 7 = cerebral cortex.

(30 min) and overnight hybridization carried out at 65°C in glass roller tubes located in an hybridization oven. After washing, the membranes were autoradiographed using Kodak X-OMAT film with intensifying screens at –80°C.

Northern analysis yielded hybridization bands between the oligonucleotide AGD probe and pineals from rats (lane 4) and steers (lane 8). It is interesting to note that the cDNA probe for AGD also hybridized to mRNA extracted from dissected blocks of rat anterior hypothalamus/preoptic area (lane 2), middle/posterior hypothalamus containing the median eminence (lane 3), and corpus striatum (lane 5). Two bands were observed, one approximately 2.4 kb and the other 0.60 kb in size. Lanes 6 and 7 are cerebellum and cerebral cortex, respectively. M_r markers were spotted in lane 1.

Northern Slot Blot of AGD mRNA Expression in Rat and Steer Pineals

A northern slot blot was also prepared (Figure 7). In this case, serial dilutions of mRNA extracted from several tissues were slot-blotted on Zeta-probe nylon membranes and hybridized with the AGD oligonucleotide probe. Hybridization intensities, evaluated with a phosphoranalyser equipped with Image Quant analysis solfware, were greatest for rat and steer pineals (lanes 2 and 5, respectively), less for the anterior hypothalamus/preoptic area (lane 3) and medial basal hypothalamus/median eminence (lane 1), and least in the corpus striatum (lane 4).

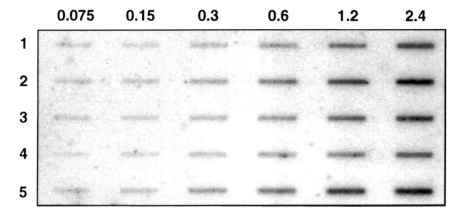

FIGURE 7

Northern slot blot analysis from AGD mRNA. Microgram amounts of tissue mRNA spotted are indicated from left to right across the top of the illustration with extracts from different tissues indicated on the left. Lane 1 = rat hypothalamic median eminence; lane 2 = rat pineal gland; lane 3 = rat anterior hypothalamus; lane 4 = rat corpus striatum; lane 5 = steer pineal gland.

Summary

The search for peptides synthesized and secreted by the pineal gland is related to early identification of the pineal gland with antigonadotropic effects and the morphology of mammalian pinealocytes which places them in the category of paraneurons.[12,13] Paraneurons are endocrine cells which secrete polypeptides in association with monoamines. Pinealocyte secretory vesicles contain serotonin, but the nature of the protein secretory products has not yet been identified..

An antigonadotropic decapeptide (AGD) has been identified in bovine pineal extracts. This neuropeptide demonstrates inhibitory effects on PRL and LH, but whether AGD represents a secretory product has not been determined. In the present study, AGD mRNA expression was observed in extracts of pineal glands and other neural tissues. This suggests that the antigonadotropic neuropeptide is synthesized in the pineal gland and may perform an autocrine or paracrine action, but its potential effect on melatonin secretion remains to be tested.

References

1. Pévet, P., Peptides in the pineal gland of vertebrates. Ultrastructural, histochemical, immunocytochemical and radioimmunological aspects, in Oksche, A. and Pévet, P., Eds., *The Pineal Organ: Photobiology-Biochronometry-Endocrinology*. Elsevier, Amsterdam, 1981, 211.

2. Ariens Kappers, J., A survey of advances in pineal research, in Reiter, R.J., Ed., *The Pineal Gland*, Vol. I, CRC Press, Boca Raton, FL, 1981, 1.

3. Benson, B., Current status of pineal peptides, *Neuroendocrinology,* 24, 241, 1977.

4. Benson, B. and Ebels, I., Other pineal peptides and related substances: physiological implications for reproductive physiology, in Reiter, R.J., Ed., *The Pineal Gland*, Vol. II, CRC Press, Boca Raton, FL, 1981, 165.

5. Vaughan, M.K., Pineal peptides: an overview, in Reiter, R.J., Ed., *The Pineal Gland,* Raven Press, New York, 1984, 39.

6. Blask, D.E., Vaughan, M.K., and Reiter, R.J., Pineal peptides and reproduction, in Relkin, R., Ed., *The Pineal Gland,* Elsevier Biomedical, New York, 1983, 201.

7. Nieuwenhuis, J.J., Arginine vasotocin (AVT), an alleged hormone of the mammalian pineal gland, *Live Sci.,* 35, 1713, 1884.

8. Benson, B., Studies on a pineal gland-derived antigonadotropic decapeptide: effects on pulsatile LH secretion in rats, *Curr. Top. Pep. Prot. Res.,* 1, 223, 1994.

9. Collin, J.-P. and Oksche, A., Structural and functional relationships in the nonmammalian pineal gland, in Reiter, R.J., Ed., *The Pineal Gland,* Vol. I, CRC Press, Boca Raton, FL, 1981, 27.

10. Lu, K.-S. and Lin, H.-S., Cytochemical studies on cytoplasmic granular elements in the hamster pineal gland, *Histochemistry,* 61, 177, 1979.

11. Pearse, A.G.E., The cytochemistry and ultrastructure of polypeptide hormone producing cells of the APUD series and the embryology, physiology and pathologic implications of the concept, *J. Histochem. Cytochem.,* 17, 303, 1969.

12. Ariens Kappers, J., Localization of indoleamine and protein synthesis in the mammalian pineal gland, in Reiter, R.J. and Wurtman, R.J., Eds., *The Pineal Gland,* Springer-Verlag, Vienna, 1978, 13.

13. Hansen, J.T. and Karasek, M., Neuron or endocrine cell? The pinealocyte as a paraneuron, in Reiter, R.J., Ed., *The Pineal Gland and Its Hormones,* Alan R. Liss, New York, 1982, 1.

14. Dwyer, V.G., Benson, B., Kwan, K.H., Humphreys, R.C., Ko, W.J., Lin, N.H., and Sammons, D.W., A computer-enhanced comparative study of brain region polypeptides and proteins by two-dimensional gel electrophoresis, *J. Pharm. Biomed. Anal.,* 6, 793, 1988.

15. Benson, B. and Ebels, I., Pineal peptides, in Reiter, R.J. and Wurtman, R.J., Eds., *The Pineal Gland,* Springer-Verlag, Vienna, 1978, 157.

16. Benson, B., Larsen, B., Findell, P.R., and Orstead, K.M., Participation of pineal peptides in reproduction, in McCann, S.M. and Dhindsa, D.S., Eds., *The Role of Peptides and Proteins in Control of Reproduction,* Elsevier, New York, 1983, 111.

17. Larsen, B.R., Findell, P.R., and Benson, B., Preliminary results — isolation and identification of pineal neurohypophysial hormone-like activity, in Reiter, R.J., Ed., *The Pineal and Its Hormones,* Alan R. Liss, New York, 1982, 117.

18. Benson, B., Ebels, I., and Hruby, V.J., Isolation and structure elucidation of bovine pineal oxytocin and an antigonadotropic peptide, in Reiter, R.J. and Lukaszyk, A., Eds., *Advances in Pineal Research,* J. Libby, London, 1990, 99.

19. Benson, B. and Ebels, I., Structure of a pineal gland-derived antigonadotropic decapeptide, *Life Sci. Phar. Lett.,* 54, PL437, 1994.

20. Benson, B. and Machen, N., Infusion of a pineal-derived antigonadotropic decapeptide into the lateral ventricle depresses prolactin levels in male rats, *Life Sci.,* 55, 263, 1994.

21. Benson, B., Pineal gland antigonadotropic decapeptide increases hypothalamic dopamine turnover, *Abstr. Exp. Biol. '97,* 3572, 619, 1997.

22. Gregory, V.M., Larsen, B., and Benson, B., Simplified HPLC-EC determination of brain catecholamines, *J. Chromat.,* 345, 140, 1985.

23. Benson, B., Machen, N., Dunn, A.M., and Wise, M.E., Chronic infusion of a pineal gland-derived antigonadotropic decapeptide alters pulsatile secretion of LH in rats, *Life Sci.,* 58, 1083, 1996.

24. Kao, C., Schaeffer, D.J., and Jackson, G.L., Different neuroendocrine systems modulate pulsatile luteinizing hormone secretion in photosuppressed and photorefractory ewes, *Biol. Reprod.,* 46, 425, 1992.

25. Dunn, A.M., Benson, B., Esquivel, E., and Wise, M.E., Threonine-rich peptide, a novel decapeptide isolated from bovine pineal glands, administered via the lateral ventricle inhibits LH release in ovariectomized ewes, *Biol. Reprod.,* 48(Suppl. 1), 91, 1993.

26. Lee, H.-J., Regulation of Hypothalamic GnRH Secretion by a Novel Decapeptide, Master's thesis, University of Arizona, Tucson, 1998.

Chapter 10

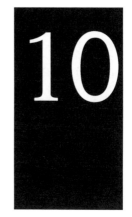

Pinoline: Formation, Distribution, and Effects

Rein Pähkla and Lembit Rägo

Contents

Introduction

The main neuroendocrine product secreted by the pineal gland is melatonin. The pharmacological effects of this pineal hormone are well characterized in a number of studies and reviews. In addition to melatonin, certain compounds of β-carboline structure can be formed in the pineal gland.

In 1961, McIsaac was first to report the formation of β-carbolines in the mammalian body as condensation products of tryptamine derivatives with aldehydes.[1] Since that time, in many laboratories these compounds have been identified as normal constituents of mammalian tissues, including those of humans. Among endogenously found β-carbolines, probably most attention has been given to the

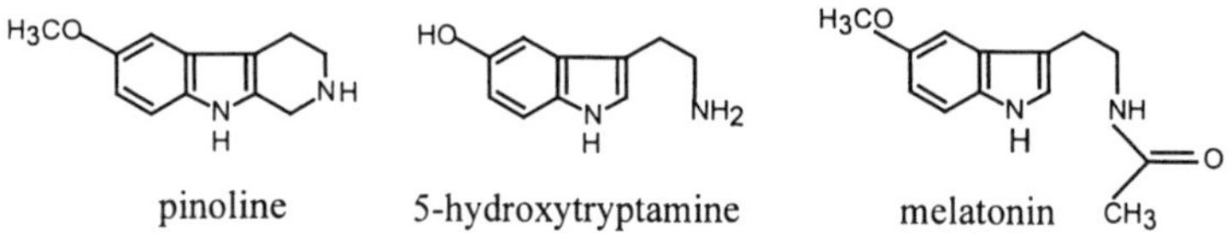

FIGURE 1
Structural formulas of pinoline, 5-hydroxytryptamine, and melatonin.

6-methoxy-1,2,3,4-tetrahydro-β-carboline (6-MeO-THBC), named "pinoline" from the words "pineal β-carboline".

Endogenous Formation of Pinoline

In animals, pinoline can enter the body directly through the diet or can be produced endogenously from dietary tryptophan via 5-hydroxytryptamine. 1,2,3,4-Tetrahydro-β-carbolines (THBCs) are easily produced from tryptamine through Pictet-Spengler condensation reaction with formaldehyde[2,3] or glyoxylic acid.[4,5] Formation of pinoline requires 5-methoxytryptamine as a substrate. 5-Methoxytryptamine is produced in the pineal gland by O-methylation of the neurotransmitter 5-hydroxytryptamine (5-HT, serotonin) by the enzyme 5-hydroxyindole-O-methyltransferase (5-HIOMT), an essential enzyme in the biosynthetic pathway of melatonin.[6,7] Therefore, endogenous synthesis of pinoline is largely confined to the pineal gland and possibly to the retina. Alternatively, pinoline can be formed from melatonin by its metabolization to 5-methoxytryptamine by the enzyme aryl acylamidase.[7,8] Structural formulas of pinoline and its possible precursors are shown in Figure 1.

The concentration of pinoline in mammalian tissues is relatively low. In 1978, Shoemaker et al.[9] localized at least one β-carboline in the rat arcuate nucleus by laser-fluorometry and suggested that it was 6-MeO-THBC. Later, Barker et al.[10] verified with mass spectrometry the presence of 6-MeO-THBC in the rat brain and adrenals and measured its concentration. The concentration of pinoline in the rat brain was 36 ng/g and in adrenal glands 1.1 µg/g. Kari and co-workers determined the concentration of pinoline in fowl pineal glands.[11,12] The concentration of pinoline was within the range of 0.11 µg/g tissue, and higher concentrations were determined during the sleep phase. Subsequently, pinoline was found to be a normal constituent in the retina of rabbits, pigs, and humans;[13,14] human serum; and cerebrospinal fluid.[15] Langer et al.[16] initially determined very high concentrations of pinoline in human postmortem pineal glands (20.6 µg/g tissue), but in later studies they were able to detect concentrations only up to 2 ng/g.[17]

A major problem in the determination of β-carbolines in biological samples is their formation during the extraction procedure. Faull et al.[18] claimed that many reported findings of β-carbolines as constituents of various tissues derive from artefactual formation of these compounds. This suggestion was supported by Bosin et al.[19] In the last 2 years, some studies have been published showing that THBCs are not present in human urine;[20,21] however, the absence of pinoline in urine does not prove the absence of this compound in serum and tissues, as most of the pinoline is metabolized in the body. In recent years, no studies have been published about the determination of pinoline levels in tissues.

Distribution and Metabolism of Pinoline

The fate of exogenously administered pinoline and other β-carbolines in animals has not been studied extensively, although the central effects of these drugs show that they are absorbed and transferred into the central nervous system. The distribution and metabolism of ^{14}C-labeled pinoline in rats was studied 26 years ago by Ho et al.[22] The results of this experiment showed that pinoline was rapidly taken up by tissues, including the brain, which had a 10 to 20 times higher concentration than blood. Pinoline was metabolized by hydroxylation of the 7 position and by demethylation of the 6-methoxy group. These metabolites were excreted into the urine, primarily as sulfate conjugates.

A whole-body autoradiographic experiment in mice by Leino et al.[23] also showed that intravenously administered [14C]pinoline was taken up by different organs. The highest concentrations of labeling were seen in kidneys, adrenal glands, intestines, and salivary glands.

Recently, we performed a series of experiments to investigate the intracellular distribution of pinoline.[24,25] In these experiments, tritiated pinoline was administered to mice intraperitoneally and tissue samples were taken for determination of total and non-specific binding 0.5 to 4 hr after administration of the compounds. Results of these experiments demonstrated that [3H]pinoline penetrates well into all tissues studied. An interesting finding was that in all tissues a great proportion of [3H]pinoline was found in cell nuclei. Nuclear binding represented up to 50% of all labels. The other characteristic finding was that in all tissues and in all subcellular structures [3H]pinoline generally binds nonspecifically. Similar intracellular localization is characteristic to the reported localization of melatonin. Melatonin is reported to penetrate cell and nuclear membranes freely, and it may accumulate within the cell nucleus.[26,27] Melatonin has been reported to bind directly to the nuclear receptors,[28,29] and we cannot exclude the possibility that pinoline can interact at least partly with the same targets in nuclei. However, the function and pharmacological significance of pinoline's nuclear binding require further studies.

Neurochemical Effects of Pinoline

The most extensively studied and probably the most important effects of pinoline are linked to the serotonergic system in the central nervous system (CNS). Pinoline has been reported to elevate brain serotonin content by inhibiting 5-HT uptake and inhibiting the monoamine oxidase-A (MAO-A) activity.

Pinoline has been reported to inhibit the uptake of 5-HT in brain synaptosomes and in platelets. The IC_{50} (concentration required to inhibit activity by 50%) values for inhibiting the uptake of ^3H- or ^{14}C-labeled 5-hydroxytryptamine *in vitro* determined in different studies ranged from 0.3 to 1.1 μM.[30–33] The IC_{50} values for inhibiting the uptake of noradrenaline and dopamine were about 50 times higher.[30,31] The inhibition appeared to be competitive both in platelets and in brain synaptosomes.[30,31]

The 5-HT uptake site is blocked by a number of antidepressant drugs. Citalopram, imipramine, and other 5-HT uptake-inhibiting antidepressants are considered to bind in serotonin transporter to the same domain that binds 5-HT or at least to the site partly overlapping the 5-HT recognition site.[34,35] Pinoline has been shown to inhibit the [^3H]imipramine binding both in platelets and neuronal membranes with IC_{50} values of 0.1 to 0.5 μM.[16,32,33] In all studies, the inhibition has been reported to be competitive.

Pinoline also interacts competitively with the most selective 5-HT uptake inhibitor, citalopram. The IC_{50} value for inhibiting [^3H]citalopram binding in rat brain homogenates was 1.3 μM.[36] Pinoline did not have any influence on the dissociation rate of specifically bound [^3H]citalopram, and chronic injection of pinoline to rats did not affect the binding parameters of this serotonin transporter ligand. Therefore, we concluded that pinoline did not have any modulative influence on the activity of 5-HT transporter and that it interacts competitively with citalopram on the substrate recognition site of the 5-HT transporter.

Pinoline also inhibits the activity of an enzyme monoamine oxidase (MAO). There are two major isoenzymes of MAO: MAO-A and MAO-B. MAO-A preferentially metabolizes serotonin and noradrenaline, and MAO-B phenylethylamine and dopamine. Pinoline has been reported to inhibit very selectively the activity of MAO-A with IC_{50} values ranging from 1 to 9 μM.[37–39] Fernandez de Arriba et al.[40] determined the kinetic parameters of MAO inhibition produced by β-carbolines and showed that pinoline was a competitive and reversible inhibitor.

Apart from the brain serotonergic system, pinoline has been shown to have no influence on other neurotransmitter receptors. It is proposed that pinoline may have unique and specific recognition sites, at least in adrenals, pineal, and brain tissues.[8] In all autoradiographic experiments performed with labeled pinoline, adrenal and pineal (when determined) glands showed high binding density. *In vitro* binding experiments performed with [^3H]pinoline revealed binding sites in bovine pineal and adrenal glands with a K_d value of 21 nM (Reference 24, and our unpublished data). However, due to very high nonspecific binding, it was not possible to characterize these binding sites further.

Pharmacological Effects of Pinoline in Animal Experiments

Beta-carbolines have been shown to exert a wide variety of actions in animal experiments. The pattern of effects of different β-carbolines depends on the structure of the compound. There are only a few studies showing the pharmacological effects of pinoline in animal experiments.

The long-known effect shared by many β-carbolines is tremor.[3,41] This effect is characteristic of β-carbolines and dihydro-β-carbolines but is less pronounced among tetrahydro-β-carbolines.[42] In rats, pinoline has been shown not to produce tremor even after intravenous doses of 100 mg/kg.[43]

The convulsive potential of β-carbolines correlates with the binding capacity of these compounds to benzodiazepine receptors.[41,42] In mice, some convulsions have been shown to precede the death after intraperitoneal injection of lethal doses of pinoline.[44] The LD_{50} for intraperitoneal injection of pinoline to mice determined in the same study was 235 mg/kg. In comparison, the LD_{50} for intraperitoneally administered amitriptyline was 65 mg/kg, and for imipramine 90 mg/kg.[45] At doses of 100 mg/kg, pinoline has been shown to have anticonvulsant properties against audiogenic and electroconvulsive seizures in mice.[46] In this study, the anticonvulsive effect was explained by serotonergic action of pinoline. Nance and Kilbey[47] showed that pinoline reversed the sucrose preference produced in rats after brain serotonin depletion. Airaksinen et al.[44] demonstrated that pinoline antagonized the group toxicity of amphetamine in mice without any effect on noradrenaline toxicity or barbiturate sleeping time and explained this also by the serotonergic effects of the drug.

An increase in the brain 5-HT level and serotonergic effects are common to most antidepressants. Therefore, we studied the effects of pinoline in the forced swimming test developed by Porsolt.[48] The forced swimming test is considered to have the highest predictive validity of antidepressant action among animal models of depression.[49,50] Pinoline showed a dose-dependent antidepressant-like effect in the rat forced swimming test (Figure 2).[51] It also reduced the activity of rats in the open field and exerted an anxiogenic-like effect in the elevated plus-maze test. All these effects can be explained by the serotonergic action of pinoline and are in line with the behavioral effects of antidepressants.

Antioxidant Actions of Pinoline

In recent years, the antioxidative properties of melatonin have been studied quite extensively. The antioxidative properties of β-carbolines have received much less attention. There are only few published data in the literature concerning the anti- or pro-oxidative potency of β-carboline compounds. Tse et al.[52] found that harman and related β-carbolines and dihydro-β-carbolines inhibited lipid peroxidation (measured as thiobarbiturate-reactive products) in a hepatic microsomal preparation incubated with oxygen radical producing systems. Kawashima et al.[53] found that 1-aryl substituted 1,2,3,4-tetrahydro-β-carboline compounds have potent effects against lipid peroxidation.

The molecular structures of pinoline and melatonin are quite similar. Both compounds share the indole nucleus and the methoxy group at the same position. Structure-activity studies comparing the free-radical scavenging ability of melatonin

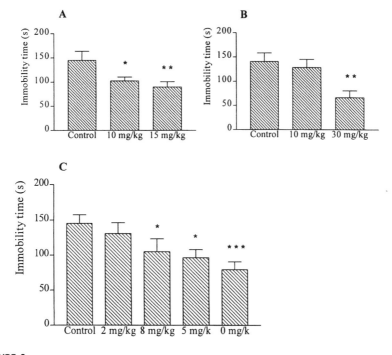

FIGURE 2

Effects of treatment with imipramine (A), amitriptyline (B), and pinoline (C) on immobility time of rats in the forced swimming test. The data are presented as mean $\pm$ SEM (n = 8). * $p < 0.05$, ** $p < 0.01$, and *** $p < 0.005$ vs. control; Fisher's PLSD test after significant ANOVA. (From Pähkla, R. et al., *Pharmacol. Res.,* 34, 73, 1996. With permission.)

with several chemically related molecules showed the importance of the methoxy group at position 5 of the indole nucleus and the *N*-acetyl group on the side chain.[54,55]

We compared the antioxidant effects of pinoline and melatonin in three different *in vitro* assay systems: the total antioxidant status determination, lipid peroxidation inhibition, and determination of the hydroxyl radical ('OH) scavenging capacity of the compounds.[56] Both compounds had comparable activity in all assay systems (Figure 3). The 'OH scavenging potency of pinoline was about 5 times lower than that of melatonin (the IC_{50} values to reduce the spin-trapping agent terephthalic acid and 'OH adduct formation were 62.3 and 11.4 µM, respectively). However, considering the fact that the 'OH scavenging ability of melatonin is possibly many times better than that of the well-known antioxidants glutathione and mannitol,[54] pinoline could still be considered a powerful 'OH scavenger. A major advantage of melatonin is its ability to penetrate into all tissues and accumulate intracellularly, particularly in the nuclei of cells.[57,58] Thus, melatonin is considered to protect nuclear DNA against radical-related damage. This protective action of melatonin is also demonstrated in *in vivo* experiments.[59] As intracellular distribution of pinoline is similar to

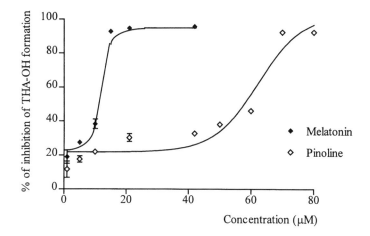

FIGURE 3

Effect of melatonin and pinoline in reducing the formation of terephthalic acid (THA)–˙OH adducts. In this experiment, hydroxyl radicals were generated via the Fenton reaction from $CuSO_4$ and H_2O_2. Generated hydroxyl radicals reacted with the THA dosimeter solution, and the reaction product was measured fluorometrically. Each point represents mean value ± SEM of 2 to 5 different determinations. (From Pähkla, R. et al., *J. Pineal Res.,* 24, 96, 1998. With permission.)

melatonin, it can be expected that pinoline at higher doses may have similar protective action against DNA oxidative damage like that of melatonin. Considering the low physiological concentrations of pinoline in the blood and in tissues, the antioxidative action is probably not the primary action of pinoline; however, in pharmacological doses, such concentrations can be reached easily.

Conclusions

Twenty years have passed since the time when pinoline was first found to be present in animal tissues; however, at this time, the physiological function and importance of this compound are not clear. Pinoline exerts mainly serotonergic effects and increases brain serotonin content by inhibiting neuronal 5-HT reuptake and its degradation by MAO. Considering the competitive interaction with serotonin, relatively low potency compared to this neurotransmitter, and low concentrations in tissues, we can suggest that modulation of brain serotonergic function is not the primary physiological action of pinoline. The nature and importance of specific pinoline binding sites require further studies. However, considering the dose-dependent, antidepressant-like behavioral effects and *in vitro* binding data combined with low toxicity and pronounced antioxidative action, this compound should be further studied as a potential antidepressant of a new pharmacological class.

References

1. McIsaac, W.M., Formation of 1-methyl-6-methoxy-1,2,3,4-tetrahydro-2-carboline under physiological conditions, *Biochem. Biophys. Acta,* 52, 607, 1961.

2. Airaksinen, M.M., and Kari, I., β-Carbolines: psychoactive compounds in the mammalian body. Part I. Occurrence, origin and metabolism, *Med. Biol.,* 59, 21, 1981.

3. Buckholtz, N.S., Neurobiology of tetrahydro-β-carbolines, *Life Sci.,* 27, 893, 1980.

4. Gynther, J., Lapinjoki, S.P., Airaksinen, M.M., and Peura, P., Decarboxylation of 1,2,3,4-tetrahydro-β-carboline-1-carboxylic acids in brain homogenate and catalysis by pyridoxal-5′-phosphate, *Biochem. Pharmacol.,* 35 2671, 1986.

5. Callaway, J.C., Gynther, J., Poso, A., Vepsalainen, J., and Airaksinen, M.M., The Pictet-Spengler reaction and biogenic tryptamines: formation of tetrahydro-β-carbolines at physiological pH, *J. Heterocyclic Chem.,* 31, 431, 1994.

6. Morton, D.J. and Potgeiter, B., Relationships between methoxyindoles and hydroxyindoles formed from 5-hydroxytryptamine in rat pineal gland, *J. Endocrinol.,* 95, 253, 1982.

7. Hardeland, R., Reiter, R.J.R., Poeggler, B., and Tan, D.-X., The significance of metabolism of the neurohormone melatonin: antioxidative protection and formation of bioactive substances, *Neurosci. Biobehav. Rev.,* 17, 347, 1993.

8. Airaksinen, M.M., Callaway, J.C., Nykvist, P., Rägo, L., Kari, E., and Gynther, J., Binding sites for [³H]pinoline, in Toitou, Y., Arendt, J., and Pévet, P., Eds., *Melatonin and the Pineal Gland — From Basic Science to Clinical Application,* Elsevier Science, New York, 1993, 83.

9. Shoemaker, D.W., Cummins, J.T., and Bidder, T.G., β-Carbolines in rat arcuate nucleus, *Neuroscience,* 3, 233, 1978.

10. Barker, S.A., Harrison, R.E., Monti, J.A., Brown, G.B., and Christian, S.T., Identification and quantification of 1,2,3,4-tetrahydro-β-carboline, 2-methyl-1,2,3,4-tetrahydro-β-carboline and 6-methoxy-1,2,3,4-tetrahydro-β-carboline as *in vivo* constituents of rat brain and adrenal gland, *Biochem. Pharmacol.,* 30, 9, 1981.

11. Kari, I., 6-Methoxy-1,2,3,4-tetrahydro-β-carboline in pineal gland of chicken and cock, *FEBS Lett.,* 127, 277, 1981.

12. Kari, I., Airaksinen, M.M., Gynther, J., and Huhtikangas, A., Mass spectrometric identification of 6-methoxy-1,2,3,4-tetrahydro-β-carboline in pineal gland, in Frigerio, A., Ed., *Recent Developments in Mass Spectrometry in Biochemistry, Medicine and Environmental Research,* Vol. 8, Elsevier, Amsterdam, 1983, 19.

13. Leino, M., Kari, I., Airaksinen, M.M., and Gynther, J., 6-Methoxy-tetrahydro-β-carboline in the retinae of rabbits and pigs, *Exp. Eye Res.,* 36, 135, 1983.

14. Leino, M., 6-Methoxy-tetrahydro-β-carboline and melatonin in the human retina, *Exp. Eye Res.,* 38, 325, 1984.

15. Rimón, R., Airaksinen, M.M., Kari, I., Gynther, J., Venäläinen, E., Heikkilä, L., Ryyppo, J., and Palo, J., Pinoline, a β-carboline derivative in the serum and cerebrospinal fluid of patients with schizophrenia, *Ann. Clin. Res.,* 16, 171, 1984.

16. Langer, S.Z., Lee, C.R., Segonzac, A., Tateishi, T., Esnaud, H., Schoemaker, H., and Winblad, B., Possible endocrine role of the pineal gland for 6-methoxytetrahydro-β-carboline, a putative endogenous neuromodulator of the [³H]imipramine recognition site, *Eur. J. Pharmacol.*, 102, 379, 1984.

17. Langer, S.Z., Galzin, A.M., Lee, C.R., and Schoemaker, H., Antidepressant-binding sites in brain and platelets, *Ciba Found. Symp.*, 123, 3, 1986.

18. Faull, K.F., Holman, R.B., Elliott, G.R., and Barchas, J.D., Tryptolines — artifact or reality: a new method of analysis using GC MS, in Bloom, F., Barchas, J., Sandler, M., and Usdin, E., Eds., *Beta-Carbolines and Tetrahydroisoquinolines. Progress in Clinical and Biological Research*, Vol. 90, Alan R. Liss, New York, 1982, 135.

19. Bosin, T.R., Holmstedt, B., Lundman, A., and Beck, O., Presence of formaldehyde in biological media and organic solvents. Artifactual formation of tetrahydro-β-carbolines, *Anal. Biochem.*, 128, 287, 1983.

20. Tsuchiya, H., Yamada, K., Todoriki, H., and Hayashi, T., Urinary excretion of tetrahydro-β-carbolines influenced by food and beverage ingestion implies their exogenous supplies via dietary sources, *J. Nutr. Biochem.*, 7 237, 1996.

21. Musshoff, F., Daldrup, T., Bonte, W., Leitner, A., and Lesch, O.M., Formaldehyde-derived tetrahydroisoquinolines and tetrahydro-β-carbolines in human urine, *J. Chromat. Biomed. Appl.*, 683, 163, 1996.

22. Ho, B.T., Taylor, D., Walker, K.E., and McIsaac, W., Metabolism of 6-methoxytetrahydro-β-carboline in rats, *Xenobiotica*, 2, 349, 1972.

23. Leino, M., Airaksinen, M.M., Antikainen, R., Gynther, J., Kari, E., Kari, I., and Peura, P., Distribution of 1,2,3,4-tetrahydro-β-carboline and 6-methoxy-1,2,3,4-tetrahydro-β-carboline in mice, *Acta Pharmacol. Toxicol.*, 54, 361, 1984.

24. Pähkla, R., Masso, R., Zilmer, M., Rägo, L., and Airaksinen, M.M., Autoradiographic localization of [³H]pinoline binding sites in mouse tissues, *Meth. Find. Exp. Clin. Pharmacol.*, 18, 359, 1996.

25. Pähkla, R., Masso, R., Rägo, L., and Airaksinen, M.M., [³H]Pinoline binding sites: autoradiographic visualization and characterization, *Acta Med. Baltica*, 3, 218, 1996.

26. Hagan, R.M. and Oakley, N.R., Melatonin comes of age?, *Trends Pharmacol. Sci.*, 16, 81, 1995.

27. Brzezinski, A., Melatonin in humans, *N. Engl. J. Med.*, 336, 186, 1997.

28. Wiesenberg, I., Missbach, M., Kahlen, J.P., Schräder, M., and Carlberg, C., Transcriptional activation of the nuclear receptor RZR alpha by the pineal gland hormone melatonin and identification of CGP 52608 as a synthetic ligand, *Nucleic Acids Res.*, 23, 327, 1995.

29. Carlberg, C., Wiesenberg, I., and Schräder, M., Nuclear signalling of melatonin, in Maestroni, G.J.M., Conti, A., and Reiter, R.J.R., Eds., *Therapeutic Potential of Melatonin. Frontiers of Hormone Research*, Vol. 3, Karger, Basel, 1997, 25.

30. Airaksinen, M.M., Svensk, H., Tuomisto, J., and Komulainen, J., Tetrahydro-β-carbolines and corresponding tryptamines: *in vitro* inhibition of serotonin and dopamine uptake by human blood platelets, *Acta Pharmacol. Toxicol.*, 46, 308, 1980.

31. Komulainen, H., Tuomisto, J., Airaksinen, M.M., Kari, I., Peura, P., and Pollari, L., Tetrahydro-β-carbolines and corresponding tryptamines: *in vitro* inhibition of serotonin, dopamine and noradrenaline uptake in rat brain synaptosomes, *Acta Pharmacol. Toxicol.*, 46, 299, 1980.

32. Langer, S.Z., Raisman, R., Tahraoui, L., Scatton, B., Niddam, R., Lee, C.R., and Claustre, Y., Substituted tetrahydro-β-carbolines are possible candidates as endogenous ligand of the [³H]imipramine recognition site, *Eur. J. Pharmacol.*, 98, 153, 1984.

33. Segonzac, A., Schoemaker, H., Tateishi, T., and Langer, S.Z., 5-Methoxytryptoline, a competitive endocoid acting at [³H]imipramine recognition sites in human platelets, *J. Neurochem.*, 45, 249, 1985.

34. Arranz, B. and Marcusson, J., [³H]Paroxetine and [³H]citalopram as markers of the brain 5-HT uptake site: a comparison study, *J. Neural Transm. (Gen. Sect.)*, 94, 27, 1994.

35. Rotondo, A., Giannaccini, G., Quattrone, C., Marazziti, D., Martini, C., Cassano, G.B., and Lucacchini, A., Solubilization and characterization of [³H]imipramine and [³H]paroxetine binding sites from calf striatum, *Neurochem. Res.*, 19, 1295, 1994.

36. Pähkla, R., Rägo, L., Callaway, J.C., and Airaksinen, M.M., Binding of pinoline on the 5-hydroxytryptamine transporter: competitive interaction with [³H]citalopram, *Pharmacol. Toxicol.*, 80, 122, 1997.

37. Meller, E., Friedman, E., Schweitzer, J.W., and Friedhoff, A., Tetrahydro-β-carbolines: specific inhibitors of type A monoamine oxidase in rat brain, *J. Neurochem.*, 28, 995, 1977.

38. Sparks, D.L. and Buckholtz, N.S., 6-Methoxy-1,2,3,4-tetrahydro-β-carboline: a specific monoamine oxidase-A inhibitor in CF-1 mouse brain, *Neurosci. Lett.*, 20, 73, 1980.

39. Glover, V., Liebowitz, J., Armando, I., and Sandler, M., β-Carbolines as selective monoamine oxidase inhibitors: *in vivo* implications, *J. Neural Trans.*, 54, 209, 1982.

40. Fernández de Arriba, A., Lizcano, J.M., Balsa, M.D., and Unzeta, M., Inhibition of monoamine oxidase from bovine retina by β-carbolines, *J. Pharm. Pharmacol.*, 46, 809, 1994.

41. Airaksinen, M.M. and Kari, I., β-Carbolines, psychoactive compounds in the mammalian body. Part II. Effects, *Med. Biol.*, 59, 190, 1981.

42. Saano, V. and Airaksinen, M.M., Binding of β-carbolines and caffeine on benzodiazepine receptors: correlations to convulsions and tremor, *Acta Pharmacol. Toxicol.*, 51, 300, 1982.

43. Airaksinen, M.M., Lecklin, A., Saano, V., Tuomisto, L., and Gynther, J., Tremorigenic effect and inhibition of tryptamine and serotonin receptor binding by β-carbolines, *Pharmacol. Toxicol.*, 60, 5, 1987.

44. Airaksinen, M.M., Ho, B.T., An, R., and Taylor, D., Major pharmacological effects of 6-methoxytetrahydro-β-carboline, a drug elevating the tissue 5-hydroxytryptamine level, *Arzneim-Forsch. Drug Res.*, 28, 42, 1978.

45. Tobe, A., Yoshida, Y., Ikoma, H., Tonomura, S., and Kikumoto, R., Pharmacological evaluation of 2-(4-methylaminobutoxy)diphenylmethane hydrochloride (MCI-2016), a new psychotropic drug with antidepressant activity, *Arzneimittel-Forschung*, 31, 1278, 1981.

46. Buckholtz, N.S., Anticonvulsant effects of 6-methoxy-1,2,3,4-tetrahydro-β-carboline on audiogenic and electroconvulsive seizures in mice, *Pharmacol. Biochem. Behav.*, 3, 65, 1975.

47. Nance, D.M. and Kilbey, M.M., Effects of dl-para-chlorophenylalanine on sucrose preference and intake: reversal by 5-hydroxytryptophan and 6-methoxy-1,2,3,4-tetrahydro-β-carboline, *Pharmacol. Biochem. Behav.*, 1, 255, 1972.

48. Porsolt, R.D., Le Pichon, M., and Jalfre, M., Depression: a new model sensitive to antidepressant treatments, *Nature*, 266, 730, 1977.

49. Willner, P., The validity of animal models of depression, *Psychopharmacology*, 83, 1, 1984.

50. Willner, P., Animal models as simulations of depression, *Trends Pharmacol. Sci.*, 12, 131, 1991.

51. Pähkla, R., Harro, J., and Rägo, L., Behavioural effects of pinoline in the rat forced swimming, open field and elevated plus-maze tests, *Pharmacol. Res.*, 34, 73, 1996.

52. Tse, S.Y., Mak, I.T., and Dickens, B.F., Antioxidative properties of harmane and beta-carboline alkaloids, *Biochem. Pharmacol.*, 42, 459, 1991.

53. Kawashima, Y., Horiguchi, A., Taguchi, M., Tuyuki, Y., Karasawa, Y., Araki, H., and Hatayama, K., Synthesis and pharmacological evaluation of 1,2,3,4-tetrahydro-β-carboline derivatives, *Chem. Pharm. Bull.*, 43, 783, 1995.

54. Tan, D.-X., Chen, L.-D., Poeggeler, B., Manchester, L.C., and Reiter, R.J.R., Melatonin: a potent, endogenous hydroxyl radical scavenger, *Endocrinol. J.*, 1, 57, 1993.

55. Scaiano, J.C., Exploratory laser flash photolysis study of free radical reactions and magnetic field effects in melatonin chemistry, *J. Pineal Res.*, 19, 189, 1995.

56. Pähkla, R., Zilmer, M., Kullisaar, T., and Rägo, L., Comparison of the antioxidant activity of melatonin and pinoline *in vitro*, *J. Pineal Res.*, 24, 96, 1998.

57. Menendez-Pelaez, A., Poeggeler, B., Reiter, R.J.R., Barlow-Walden, L.R., Pablos, M.I., and Tan, D.-X., Nuclear localization of melatonin in different mammalian tissues: immunological and radioimmunoassay evidence, *J. Cell. Biochem.*, 53, 373, 1993.

58. Reiter, R.J.R., Tan, D.-X., Poeggeler, B., Menendez-Pelaez, A., Chen, L.-D., and Saarela, S., Melatonin as a free radical scavenger: implications for aging and age-related diseases, *Ann. N.Y. Acad. Sci.*, 719, 1, 1994.

59. Reiter, R.J.R., Antioxidant actions of melatonin, *Adv. Pharmacol.*, 38, 103, 1997.

Chapter

Melatonin and Cancer Treatment

Paolo Lissoni

Contents

Introduction

Until a few years ago, the attention of oncologists had been limited to the analysis of tumor biological characteristics, including histology and genetic properties. In contrast, very little time was spent investigating the immuno-endocrine status of cancer patients, who have been simply considered tumor-bearing subjects, without

0-8493-8564-4/99/$0.00+$.50
© 1999 by CRC Press LLC

researching a possible explanation for the neoplastic progression in their immune and neuroendocrine status.

After the discovery of interleukins (IL), great advances have been achieved in the knowledge of antitumor immunity, and at present the immune status of cancer patients is included within the prognostic factors influencing the clinical history of the neoplastic disease.[1] Today, it is known that the activation of an effective anticancer immune reaction depends on complex feedback mechanisms operating among cytokines. IL-2, which is produced by T helper-type 1 lymphocytes (Th1),[2] and IL-12,[3] mainly released by macrophages, represent the two main antitumor cytokines in humans. IL-6[4] and IL-10[5] would constitute the main cytokines responsible for macrophage-mediated and T helper-type 2 lymphocyte (Th2)-induced suppression of host anticancer immunity, respectively. The most important cytotoxic cells involved in determining cancer cell destruction are lymphokine-activated killer (LAK) cells, which originate from natural killer (NK) cells, and T cytotoxic lymphocytes (CD8), primarily activated by IL-2 and by IL-12, respectively.[1,6] In addition, recent advances in the knowledge of neuroimmunomodulation (NIM) have demonstrated that the *in vivo* immune responses are physiologically under a central neuroendocrine control, mainly exerted by the opioid system[7] and by the pineal gland.[8] The opioid system would play an immunosuppresive role,[7] whereas several pineal substances have been proven to stimulate the immune system in an antitumor way.[8] At present, the indole melatonin (MLT) represents the most investigated pineal hormone provided by both oncostatic and immunomodulatory activities.[8,9] MLT secretion shows a circadian rhythm, with lowest values during the day and highest blood concentrations during the dark period of the night.[10] The existence of a normal light/dark rhythm of MLT has appeared to be essential for maintaining optimal immune performance.[9] In addition, surgical[11] or chemical[9] pinealectomy has been shown to suppress IL-2-dependent antitumor immune reactions. The evidence of MLT circadian rhythm constitutes a fundamental biological marker of the status of health,[10] and alterations in MLT rhythm have been documented in several human diseases, including cancer.[8,10] The lack of a physiological nocturnal increase would represent the most frequently described alteration of MLT rhythm.[10]

The Biochemistry of Cancer Growth

At present, it is known that cancer cell proliferation depends on several factors, including genetic characteristics of cancer cells responsible for the degree of biological malignancy, production of tumor growth factors by cancer cells themselves or by host biological systems, and host anticancer immune defenses. Several immune alterations have been observed in advanced cancer patients involving both number and function of immune cells, as well as the endogenous production of cytokines. Cancer-related cytokine alterations are characterized by an altered balance between suppressive and immunostimulating cytokines, with a shift toward a preferential production of immunosuppressive cytokines, such as IL-6 and IL-10,[12] whereas the endogenous secretion of the antitumor cytokine IL-2 tends to decrease progressively with the progression of the neoplastic disease.[13] Advanced cancer patients are also characterized by psychoneuroendocrine alterations, mainly involving the pineal function,[8] and it has been suggested that cancer-related immune alterations would depend at least in part on changes in the psychoneuroendocrine system, rather than being due to primary damage of the immune cells themselves.[14] Therefore, cancer onset and progression would represent at least in part the effect of a systemic disorder, mainly involving psychoneuroendocrine and immune systems.

Antitumor Mechanisms of Melatonin

For more than 50 years, it has been known that the pineal gland plays an antitumor physiological role,[8] whereas most other endocrine glands tend to stimulate tumor progression, including hypophysis, gonads, and adrenal glands. Moreover, it has been known for more than 20 years that MLT may induce objective tumor regression in animals,[8,15] even though it is not the only pineal substance responsible for the anticancer action of the pineal gland. However, only recent advances in the knowledge of the immunobiology of tumors have allowed us to explain the mechanism responsible for the antitumor activity of MLT. At present, the oncostatic action of MLT is considered to depend on four main mechanisms involving cancer cells themselves and host immune reactivity:

1. *Possible direct cytostatic action.* MLT has appeared to inhibit the growth of some cancer cell lines *in vitro,* primarily breast cancer and melanoma.[15] The effects of MLT on the proliferation of normal and neoplastic cells are very controversial, as it has been shown either to inhibit or to stimulate cell proliferation. These apparently contradictory results may be explained by the recently acquired knowledge concerning the action of MLT in the modulation of the apoptotic process (e.g., programmed cell death).[16] MLT would influence the apoptosis by acting on specific nuclear melatoninergic receptors involved in the regulation of oncogene and anti-oncogene expression, and it would be able either to inhibit the apoptosis in the presence of an enhanced apoptotic process, such as in bone marrow hypoplasia, or to reinduce the apoptosis in the case of a loss of apoptosis itself, such as in the neoplastic transformation.

2. *Inhibition of tumor growth factor production.* The growth of most tumor histotypes would require the presence of particular growth factors. Prolactin (PRL) is a growth factor for breast cancer and prostate cancer. Melanocyte-stimulating hormone (MSH) is a growth factor for melanoma. Growth hormone (GH), insulin-like growth factor-1 (IGF-1), and epidermal growth factor (EGF) have been shown to stimulate the growth of several cancer histotypes, including lung cancer, gastrointestinal tumors, breast cancer, prostate cancer, and endocrine tumors. MLT may inhibit and/or modulate the production of several tumor growth factors, including PRL, GH, MSH, IGF-1, and EGF.[8,10,15,16]

3. *Differentiation of cancer cells.* It is known that the differentiation of tumor cells, including their hormone dependency, is related to oncogene and antioncogene expression.

MLT has been proven to stimulate endocrine receptor expression on cancer cells, primarily breast cancer,[8,15] with a subsequent increase in hormone dependency of cancer cells and a decrease in their biological malignancy.

4. *Stimulation of host anticancer immune defenses.* The pineal gland would represent a target organ for cytokine action, and it would play a physiological central regulatory role in peripheral feedback mechanisms operating among cytokines.[17] The recent advances in the immunology of cytokines have allowed us to better define the immunomodulatory role of MLT on host anticancer defenses.

Mechanisms of the Stimulatory Role of Melatonin on Anticancer Immunity

It has been demonstrated that cancer cell lysis is mediated by LAK cells and CD8[+]-T lymphocytes[1] by a non-major histocompatibility complex (MHC)-restricted and a MHC-restricted cytotoxic mechanism, respectively. Eosinophils activated by IL-5 also play an antitumor role through the release of cytotoxic proteins.[1] In contrast, macrophages would mediate the suppression of antitumor cytotoxicity by secreting several substances capable of inhibiting IL-2-dependent anticancer activity, including IL-6, prostaglandin E2 (PgE2), nitric oxide (NO), and IL-10.[18] Macrophages may also exert an antitumor action by producing IL-12.[19] IL-15, produced by macrophages, is also able to induce antitumor effects, and its activity would be similar to that of IL-2 in terms of mechanisms of action.[20] It is also known that Th lymphocytes may differentiate into Th1 or Th2 under the action of IL-12 or IL-4, respectively. The preferential differentiation into Th2 would stimulate cancer growth through the release of IL-10, which may inhibit IL-2 secretion and activity, as well as the secretion of IL-12.[21] IL-4, also produced by Th2 cells, would determine a main stimulatory effect on cancer growth, either by counteracting IL-2-induced LAK cell generation, or by promoting Th differentiation into Th2 cells.[22] In contrast, Th2 production of IL-5 would have a favorable prognostic significance because of its potential capacity of generating antitumor eosinophils.[1]

The enhanced differentiation into Th2 cells and the hyperactivation of macrophages in a suppressive way seem to represent the primary mechanisms responsible for the lack of an effective anticancer immune response in cancer patients. MLT has been proven to amplify IL-2 secretion by acting on specific melatonin receptors expressed on Th1 lymphocytes,[23] to reduce IL-6 secretion in basal conditions,[24] to inhibit IL-10 release in response to IL-2,[24] and to stimulate macrophage production of IL-12 in the presence of IL-2, whereas IL-2 alone has no relevant stimulatory action on IL-12 release.[25] Therefore, MLT would stimulate anticancer immunity by promoting differentation of Th1 lymphocytes, with subsequent enhanced production of IL-2, and by inhibiting macrophage-mediated suppressive events in response to IL-2, as well as Th2 cell-mediated immunosuppression. In other words, MLT would exert antitumor immunomodulatory effects by piloting in an antitumor way the great variety of cytokine effects induced by IL-2 and IL-12, either by inhibiting macrophage- and

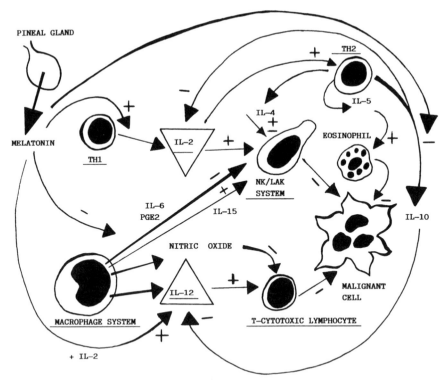

FIGURE 1

Cytokine interactions in generating the antitumor immune response and their modulation by the pineal hormone melatonin.

Th2-mediated immunosuppression or by enhancing the endogenous production of IL-2 and IL-12. The immunomodulatory effects of MLT on host anticancer immunity are illustrated in the Figure 1.

Clinical Protocols With Melatonin in Oncology: General Considerations

It would be a great mistake to imagine MLT therapy of cancer as being in opposition to classical antitumor treatment. MLT therapy does not oppose, but rather integrates, conventional medical therapies of cancer according to a new biological and systemic philosophy of the neoplastic disease. First, we have to take into consideration that almost all drugs commonly used in the medical treatment of cancer may act through one of the following mechanisms: (1) direct cytotoxic or cytostatic action, (2) differentation of cancer cells, (3) inhibition of tumor growth factors and/or angiogenetic factors, and (4) stimulation of host anticancer immunity. MLT would represent perhaps the only biological substance known up to now which is capable of exerting all potential antitumor mechanisms commonly involved in the classical medical oncology.

The first studies of MLT in the treatment of human neoplasms were performed in 1970 by Starr et al.,[26] who reported promising clinical results in patients affected by advanced sarcomas. Following their research, no other clinical study of MLT was published until the later reports by Monza Hospital. MLT therapy for cancer was also investigated by Di Bella et al.,[27] but unfortunately no clinical trial was published by them.

In animals, MLT has been proven to induce objective tumor regression only when given at pharmacological doses and during the dark period of the day.[8] The clinical protocols with MLT in the treatment of advanced cancer patients were designed on the basis of the aforementioned experimental evidence (e.g., high-dose MLT and evening administration). The sequence of Monza's studies with MLT in human neoplasms recognized six different phases: (1) MLT alone in the palliative therapy of untreatable cancer patients; (2) MLT plus cytokines, primarily IL-2; (3) MLT plus classical endocrine therapy; (4) MLT plus chemoterapy; (5) MLT plus radiotherapy (RT); and (6) MLT as adjuvant endocrine therapy.

The efficacy of MLT was evaluated according to World Health Organization criteria. Complete response (CR) was defined as a complete regression of all neoplastic lesions for at least 1 month; partial response (PR) was defined as a reduction of at least 50% in the sum of the products of the longest perpendicular diameters for at least 1 month; stable disease (SD) was no objective cancer regression or increase greater than 25%; progressive disease (PD) was an increase of at least 25% in measurable lesions or the appearance of new lesions. Moreover, most advanced solid tumor patients treated with MLT at Monza Hospital had an expected survival time lower than 12 months.

Melatonin Alone in the Palliative Therapy of Untreatable Solid Tumor Patients

One study, undertaken in 1985[28] included 200 untreatable metastatic solid tumor patients for whom no other effective standard therapy was available and whose life expectancy was less than 6 months. MLT was given orally at 20 mg/day in the evening, every day, until disease progression. No patient had a CR. A PR was achieved in 5 patients only (2.5%). SD was obtained in 82/200 (41%) patients. Moreover, a survival longer than 1 year was achieved in 38/200 (16%) patients. No apparent MLT-related toxicity occured; to the contrary, several patients experienced an improved quality of life. In particular, MLT was effective in the relief of asthenia, anxiety, cachexia, and depression. The characteristics of patients and their clinical results are shown in Table 1.

TABLE 1
Clinical Data and Response to Therapy in 200 Untreatable Metastatic Solid Tumor Patients Receiving MLT[a] as Palliative Treatment

Histotype	No.	CR	PR	SD	Survival At 1 Year
Overall patients	200	0	5	82	38
Lung cancer	81	0	1	40	18
NSCLC[c]	77	0	1	39	17
SCLC[c]	4	0	0	1	1
Colon cancer	36	0	1	9	5
Breast cancer	16	0	0	7	1
Gastric cancer	12	0	0	5	2
Renal cell cancer	12	0	1	5	4
Pancreatic cancer	11	0	1	4	2
Sarcoma	9	0	0	4	3
Hepatocarcinoma	8	0	1	4	2
Gynecologic tumors	8	0	0	2	0
Testis cancer	4	0	0	0	0
Melanoma	3	0	0	2	1

Clinical Response (WHO)[b] spans CR, PR, SD columns.

[a] 20mg/day orally in the evening.

[b] CR = complete response; PR = partial response; SD = stable disease.

[c] NSCLC = non-small-cell lung cancer; SCLC = small-cell lung cancer.

Cancer Neuroimmunotherapy With Melatonin and Antitumor Cytokines

Cancer neuroimmunotherapy is defined as a concomitant administration of antitumor cytokines, such as IL-2, and neuroimmunomodulating agents, such as MLT, in an attempt to reproduce the physiological links existing between neurohormones and cytokines. *In vivo,* it is known that the immune responses depend not only on the activity of the immune cells, but also on a central regulation played by neurohormones and neuropeptides. Chemical or surgical pinealectomy has appeared to reduce IL-2 secretion and activity. Because of the evidence of alterations of the MLT light/dark rhythm,[8] the pineal status of advanced cancer patients could be comparable to that of a functional pinealectomy. Therefore, in this condition, the antitumor efficacy of IL-2 administration would be diminished, and it is probable that the induction of a normal pineal function by an exogenous administration of MLT during the dark period of the day could enhance IL-2 efficacy in the immunotherapy of cancer. This is the primary rationale for the MLT association with anticancer cytokines. In fact, our previous clinical studies demonstrated that MLT may reduce IL-2 toxicity and amplify its therapeutic results in advanced solid tumors generally resistant to IL-2 alone.[28] The schedule of cancer neuroimmunotherapy with subcutaneous, low-dose IL-2 plus MLT was as follows: IL-2 at 3 million IU/day in the evening for 6 days/ week for 4 consecutive weeks, corresponding to one complete immunotherapeutic cycle, in association with MLT at 40 mg/day orally in the evening every day. In non-progressing patients, a second cycle was given after a 21-day rest period; then, patients underwent a maintenance period consisting of 1 week of therapy every month until disease progression. At present, the data include 320 locally advanced or metastatic solid tumor patients with life expectancy less than 6 months and for whom no other effective standard therapy was available. The clinical results are reported in Table 2. Most patients were suffering from non-small-cell lung cancer and gas-trointestinal tract tumors. Objective tumor regression was achieved in 53/320 (17%) patients, and non-small cell lung cancer, hepatocarcinoma, pancreatic adenocarci-noma, gastric cancer, and endocrine tumors were the most responsive neoplasms, either in terms of regression rate or survival time. The toxicity was low in most cases, as side-effects were generally limited to episodes of fever of less than 39°C during the first days of IL-2 injection, and most patients received the treatment as a home therapy.

Long-term results with low-dose subcutaneous IL-2 plus MLT in advanced cancer patients with life expectancy less than 6 months showed 3-year survival in about 9% of the patients,[29] which was significantly higher with respect to both supportive care or IL-2 alone. Therefore, the neuroimmunotherapy with low-dose IL-2 plus MLT could constitute one of the most effective treatments available up to now in the treatment of hepatocarcinoma, cancer of the pancreas, and advanced non-small-cell lung cancer. In particular, in a randomized study in advanced non-small-cell lung cancer, low-dose IL-2 plus MLT has been shown to induce a tumor regression rate comparable to that obtained with chemotherapy with cisplatin plus etoposide, but with a significantly longer survival.[30]

Melatonin Plus Classical Endocrine Therapy

Several reports have suggested that MLT may enhance the hormone dependency of tumors[8] by stimulating endocrine receptor expression and modulating oncogene activation. The concomitant administration of MLT (20 mg/day orally in the evening, every day until progression) has appeared to reverse the clinical resistance to the classical endocrine therapy of metastatic breast cancer[31] and metastatic prostate cancer[32] treated, respectively, with the anti-estrogen tamoxifen and LHRH analogs in about 20% of the patients. Moreover, the neuroendocrine combination of MLT (20 mg/day orally in the evening) plus tamoxifen (20 mg/day orally at noon) has been shown to be effective in several tumor histotypes other than classical hormone-dependent tumors (e.g., breast cancer and prostate cancer).[33] Because of its absolute

TABLE 2
Clinical Results in Relation to Tumor Histotype of Neuroimmunotherapy With Low-Dose IL-2 plus Melatonin in 320 Untreatable Advanced Solid Tumor Patients With Life Expectancy Less than 6 Months

| Histotype | No. | Clinical Response (WHO)[a] | | | | Survival At 1 Year |
		CR	PR	OR (%)	SD	No. (%)
Overall tumors	320	4	49	53 (17%)	149	128 (40%)
Lung cancer						
NSCLC[b]	71	0	13	13 (18%)	39	29 (40%)
SCLC[b]	4	0	0	0	1	1 (25%)
Gastrointestinal tumors						
Pancreatic cancer	38	1	3	4 (11%)	14	10 (26%)
Hepatocarcinoma	32	2	8	10 (31%)	15	18 (56%)
Colorectal carcinoma	31	0	4	4 (13%)	11	10 (32%)
Gastric cancer	26	1	5	6 (23%)	11	11 (42%)
Biliary tract tumors	8	0	1	1 (13%)	3	2 (25%)
Breast cancer	15	0	2	2 (13%)	5	4 (27%)
Endocrine tumors	14	0	4	4 (29%)	6	8 (57%)
Gynecologic tumors	14	0	2	2 (14%)	6	5 (36%)
Pleural mesothelioma	14	0	1	1 (7%)	9	5 (36%)
Soft tissue sarcomas	13	0	1	1 (8%)	8	6 (46%)
Renal cell cancer	12	0	2	2 (17%)	8	8 (67%)
Melanoma	10	0	1	1 (10%)	4	3 (30%)
Prostate cancer	8	0	1	1 (13%)	4	4 (50%)
Head and neck cancers	4	0	1	1 (25%)	2	3 (75%)
Unknown primary tumors	3	0	0	0	1	0 (0%)
Osteosarcoma	3	0	0	0	2	1 (33%)

[a] CR = complete response; PR = partial response; OR = overall response; SD = stable disease.

[b] NSCLC = non-small-cell lung cancer; SCLC = small-cell lung cancer.

tolerability, this schedule of treatment could represent a possible effective therapy of advanced solid tumor patients in a poor clinical status, regardless of sites of disease and tumor histotype. Therefore, this proposed therapy could allow us to eliminate the statement that "there is nothing we can do" which is often pronounced by the oncologists for advanced cancer patients of poor clinical condition; this therapy could also allow us to abrogate the separation between palliative and curative therapies of cancer. The potential efficacy of the MLT/tamoxifen association would be related to some biological properties of tamoxifen other than its anti-estrogenic action, particularly the stimulation of transforming growth factor-beta (TGF-β) secretion, which plays a cytostatic action against several cancer histotypes. Unfortunately, TGF has an important immunosuppressive effect that would be counteracted by the immuno-enhancing action of MLT.

Melatonin Plus Cancer Chemotherapy

Despite its capacity for inducing objective tumor regression, chemotherapy has not been proven to prolong the survival time in several tumor histotypes, including non-small-cell lung cancer, hepatocarcinoma, cancer of the pancreas, and biliary tract cancers. These findings are dependent upon the extent of chemotherapy-induced damage of the immune system which plays a relevant role in influencing the clinical history of the neoplastic disease. Experimental studies have shown that MLT may abrogate chemotherapy-induced bone marrow and immune damage.[34] Moreover, MLT has appeared to be a potent scavenger of oxygen free radicals, which are involved in mediating the toxicity of both chemotherapy and RT.[35] These experimental data constitute the rationale of MLT-chemotherapy association. In a randomized study,[36] MLT has been shown to reduce the toxicity of various chemotherapeutic agents, including cisplatin, etoposide, anthracyclines, and 5-fluorouracil. In particular, MLT has appeared to be effective in preventing chemotherapy-induced thrombocytopenia, stomatitis, neurotoxicity, asthenia, cachexia, and psychogenic vomiting, whereas vomiting and alopecia were not reduced by MLT. In addition, in advanced non-small-cell lung cancer and gastrointestinal tract cancer patients of poor clinical status treated with cisplatin plus etoposide and with 5-fluorouracil plus folates,[37,38] respectively, the concomitant administration of MLT (20 mg/day orally in the evening every day) has appeared to enhance both tumor response rate and survival time. According to these results, at present the decision to administer chemotherapeutic drugs without MLT would have to be considered sadistic, as it could deprive the patients of a simple, economic, and nontoxic therapy which is more effective than cancer chemotherapy alone.

Melatonin Plus Radiotherapy

As mentioned before, RT-induced toxicity and immune damage may be reduced by MLT, probably by counteracting RT-induced generation of oxygen free radicals,[35] which play a role in determining RT-related genetic damage. Because MLT would represent the most effective antioxidant agent known up to now, the use of MLT in association with RT seems to be justified. In fact, preliminary results in glioblastoma patients would suggest that MLT may improve the quality of life and the survival time compared to RT alone.[39]

TABLE 3
Percent of Disease-Free Survival in Surgically Treated Cancer Patients at High Risk for Recurrence Undergoing Adjuvant Therapy of Melatonin[a] or No Treatment After a Median Followup of 25 Months

Histotype	Melatonin Group		No Treatment	
	No.	Disease-Free Survival (%)	No.	Disease-Free Survival (%)
Node positive lung cancer	11	8 (73%)[b]	9	3 (33%)
Node postive gastric cancer	16	11 (69%)[b]	14	5 (36%)
Node relapsed melanoma	14	7 (50%)[b]	16	2 (12%)

[a] 20 mg/day orally.

[b] $p < 0.05$ vs. controls.

Melatonin as Adjuvant Endocrine Therapy

Adjuvant chemotherapy has been evaluated in several surgically treated solid tumor patients at high risk for recurrence because of node involvement at the time of surgical removal of the primary tumor. However, adjuvant chemotherapy has clearly been shown to be effective in prolonging disease-free survival in breast cancer and perhaps colon cancer patients. Again, this finding could depend on the extent of chemotherapy-induced immune damage. Because of its potential antiproliferative action and immunostimulating effect, MLT could be investigated as an adjuvant therapy. As shown in Table 3, preliminary (unpublished) data in node-involved melanoma, lung cancer, and gastric cancer patients would suggest that MLT adjuvant therapy (20 mg/day orally in the evening until disease recurrence) may prolong the disease-free period.

Other Indications of Melatonin in Medical Oncology

MLT has appeared to enhance the antitumor efficacy of IL-2 and to reduce its toxicity.[28] As far as the association with cytokines other than IL-2 is concerned, preliminary studies showed that melatonin may reduce the toxicity of tumor necrosis factor-alpha (TNF-α), mainly thrombocytopenia and hypotension, and of interferon-alpha, particulary asthenia and depression,[40] while no conclusion may be drawn as to the possible influence of MLT on the antitumor efficacy of cytokines other than IL-2.

Melatonin has been proven to improve the hematological status of patients with myelodysplastic syndrome secondary to cancer chemotherapy, and a survival rate of about 4 years in 2/6 patients was achieved. Such a long survival time has perhaps never been described in patients with secondary myelodysplastic syndrome.[41] Finally, high-dose MLT alone has been shown to induce objective tumor regression in more than 10% of melanomas resistant to chemotherapy.[42]

Conclusions

Melatonin may represent a very useful drug in medical oncology, either alone as a palliative therapy for untreatable cancer patients, or in association with IL-2 to enhance its antitumor efficacy, with classical endocrine therapy to reverse the clinical resistance, and with chemotherapy and RT to reduce their toxicity and perhaps to prolong the survival time. Further studies are required to establish whether MLT efficacy depends on the expression of MLT receptors on cancer cells and on an altered MLT circadian rhythm prior to therapy.

References

1. Atzpodien, J. and Kirchner, H., Cancer, cytokines and cytotoxic cells: interleukin-2 in the immunotherapy of human neoplasms, *Klin.Wochenschr.*, 68, 1, 1990.

2. Rosenberg, S.A., The immunotherapy and gene therapy of cancer, *J. Clin. Oncol.*, 10, 180, 1992.

3. Banks, R.E., Patel, P.M., and Selby, P.J., Interleukin-12: a new clinical player in cytokine therapy, *Br. J. Cancer*, 71, 655, 1995.

4. Kishimoto, T., The biology of interleukin-6, *Blood*, 74, 1, 1989.

5. Moore, K.W., O'Garra, A., De Waal-Malefyt, R., Vieira, P., and Mosmann, T.R., Interleukin-10, *Ann. Rev. Immunol.*, 11, 165, 1993.

6. Wigginton, J.M., Komschlies, K.L., Back, T.C., Franco, J.L., Brunda, M.J., and Wiltrout, R.H., Administration of interleukin 12 with pulse interleukin-2 and the rapid and complete eradication of murine renal carcinoma, *J. Natl. Cancer Inst.*, 88, 38, 1996.

7. Manfredi, B., Sacerdote, P., Bianchi, M., Locatelli, L., Velijc-Radulovic, J., and Panerai, A.E., Evidence for an opioid inhibitory tone on T-cell proliferation, *J. Neuroimmunol.*, 44, 43, 1993.

8. Regelson, W. and Pierpaoli, W., Melatonin: a rediscovered antitumor hormone?, *Cancer Invest.*, 5, 379, 1987.

9. Maestroni, G.J.M., The immunoeuroendocrine role of melatonin, *J. Pineal Res.*, 14, 1, 1993.

10. Arendt, J., Melatonin, *Clin. Endocrinol.*, 29, 205, 1988.

11. Del Gobbo, V., Libri, V., Villani, N., Calio, R., and Nistico, G., Pinealectomy inhibits interleukin-2 production and natural killer activity in mice, *Int. J. Immunopharmacol.*, 11, 567, 1989.

12. Clerici, M. and Clerici, E., The tumor enhancement phenomenon: reinterpretation from Th1/Th2 perspective, *J. Natl. Cancer Inst.*, 88, 461, 1996.

13. Lissoni, P., Barni, S., Rovelli, F., and Tancini, G., Lower survival in metastatic cancer patients with reduced interleukin-2 blood concentrations. Preliminary report, *Oncology*, 48, 125, 1991.

14. Lissoni, P., Barni, S., Cattaneo, G., Archili, C., Rovelli, F., Rescaldani, R., Brivio, F., Pelizzoni, F., Esposti, D., De Martini, G., Scaglione, F., and Fraschini, F., Pineal-interleukin-2 interactions and their possible importance in the pathogenesis of immune dysfunctions in cancer, *Life Sci.*, 204, 273, 1991.

15. Bartsch, C., Bartsch, H., and Lippert, T.H., The pineal gland and cancer: facts, hypoteses and perspectives, *Cancer J.*, 5, 194, 1992.

16. Cos, S. and Blask, D.E., Melatonin modulates growth factor activity in MCF-7 human breast cancer cells, *J. Pineal Res.*, 17, 25, 1994.

17. Lissoni, P., Tisi, E., Brivio, F., Ardizzoia, A., Crispino, S., Barni, S., Tancini, G., Conti, A., and Maestroni, G.J.M., Modulation of interleukin-2-induced macrophage activation in cancer patients by the pianeal hormone melatonin, *J. Biol. Regul. Homeost. Agents*, 5, 154, 1991.

18. Alleva, D.G., Burger, C.J., and Elgert, K.D., Tumor-induced regulation of suppressor macrophage nitric oxide and TNF-alpha production, *J. Immunol.*, 153, 1674, 1994.

19. Wigginton, J.M., Kuhns, D.B., Back, T.C., Brunda, M.J., Wiltrout, R.H., and Cox, G.W., Interleukin 12 primes macrophage for nitric oxide production *in vivo* and in tumor-bearing mice: implications for the antitumor activity of interleukin 12 and/or interleukin 2, *Cancer Res.*, 56, 1131, 1996.

20. Gamero, A.M., Ussery, D:, Reintgen, D.S., Puleo, C.A.. and Djeu, J.Y., Interleukin-15 induction of lymphokine-activated killer cell function against CD18-dependent, perforin-related mechanism, *Cancer Res.*, 55, 4988, 1995.

21. Swain, S.L., Weinberg, A.D., English, M., and Huston, G., IL-4 directs the development of Th2-like helper effectors, *J. Immunol.*, 145, 3796, 1990.

22. Paul, W.E., Inteleukin-4: a prototypic immunoregulatory lymphokine, *Blood*, 77, 1859, 1991.

23. Gonzales-Haba, M.G., Garcia-Maurino, S., Calvo, J.R., Goberna, R., and Guerrero, J.M., High-affinity binding of melatonin by human circulating T lymphocytes (CD4+), *FASEB J.*, 9, 1331, 1995.

24. Lissoni, P., Pittalis, S., Rovelli, F., Vigorè, L., Roselli, M.G., and Brivio, F., Interleukin-2, melatonin and interleukin-12 as a possible neuroimmune combination in the biotherapy of cancer, *J. Biol. Regul. Homeost. Agents*, 9, 63, 1995.

25. Lissoni, P., Pittalis, S., Brivio, F., Rovelli, F., and Pelizzoni, F., Modulation of IL-2-IL-12 relation by the pineal gland, *Eur. Cytokine Netw.*, 7, 542, 1996.

26. Starr, K.W., Growth and new growth: environmental carcinogens in the process of human ontogeny, *Prog. Clin. Cancer*, 4, 1, 1970.

27. Di Bella, L., Rossi, M.T., and Scalera, G., Perspectives in pineal functions, *Prog. Brain Res.*, 52, 475, 1979.

28. Lissoni, P., Barni, S., Tancini, G., Ardizzoia, A., Ricci, G., Aldeghi, R., Brivio, F., Tisi, E., Rovelli, F., Rescaldani, R., Quadro, G., and Maestroni, G.J.M., A randomised study with subcutaneous low-dose interleukin-2 alone vs. interleukin-2 plus the pineal neurohormone melatonin in advanced solid neoplasm other than renal cancer and melanoma, *Br. J. Cancer*, 69, 196, 1994.

29. Lissoni, P., Laudon, M., Barni, S., Brivio, F., Tisi, E., Rovelli, F., Chatikhine, V., Fumagalli, L., Maestroni, G., Conti, A., and Tancini, G., Long-term results of cancer immunotherapy with subcutaneous low-dose interleukin-2 plus melatonin, *Int. J. Immunother.* (in press).

30. Lissoni, P., Meregalli, S., Fossati, V., Paolorossi, F., Barni, S., Tancini, G., and Frigerio, F., A randomized study of immunotherapy with low-dose subcutaneous interleukin-2 plus melatonin vs. chemotherapy with cisplatin and etoposide as first-line therapy for advanced non-small cell lung cancer, *Tumori*, 80, 464, 1994.

31. Lissoni, P., Barni, S., Meregalli, S., Fossati, V., Cazzaniga, M., Esposti, D., and Tancini, G., Modulation of cancer endocrine therapy by melatonin: a phase II study of tamoxifen plus melatonin in metastatic breast cancer patients progressing under tamoxifen alone, *Br. J. Cancer*, 71, 854, 1995.

32. Lissoni, P. Cazzaniga, M., Tancini, G., Scardino, E., Musci, R., Barni, S., Maffezzini, M., Meroni, T., Rocco, F., Conti, A., and Maestroni, G.J.M., Reversal of clinical resistance to LHRH-analogue in metastatic prostate cancer by the pineal hormone melatonin, *Eur. Urol.*, 31, 178, 1997.

33. Lissoni, P., Paolorossi, F., Tancini, G., Ardizzoia, A., Barni, S., Brivio, F., Maestroni, G.J.M., and Chilelli, M., A phase II study of tamoxifen plus melatonin in metastatic tumor patients, *Br. J. Cancer*, 74, 1466, 1996.

34. Maestroni, G.J.M., Conti, A., and Lissoni, P., Colony-stimulating activity and hematopoietic rescue from cancer chemotherapy compounds are induced by melatonin via endogenous interleukin-4, *Cancer Res.*, 54, 4740, 1994.

35. Poeggeler, B., Reiter, R.J., Tan, D.X., Chen, L.D., and Manchester, L.C., Melatonin, hydroxyl radical-mediated oxidative damage, and aging: a hypothesis, *J. Pineal Res.*, 14, 151, 1993.

36. Lissoni, P., Tancini, G., Barni, S., Paolorossi, F., Ardizzoia, A., Conti, A., and Maestroni, G.J.M., Treatment of cancer chemotherapy-induced toxicity with the pineal hormone melatonin, *Supp. Care Cancer*,5, 212, 1997.

37. Lissoni, P., Paolorossi, F., Ardizzoia, A., Barni, S., Chilelli, M., Mancuso, M., Tancini, G., Conti , A., and Maestroni, G.J.M., A randomized study of chemotherapy with cisplatin, etoposide and the pineal hormone melatonin as a first line treatment of advanced non-small cell lung cancer patients in a poor clinical status, *J. Pineal Res.*, 23, 15, 1997.

38. Lissoni, P., Barni, S., Paolorossi, F., Ardizzoia, A., Ricci, G., Chilelli, M., and Tancini, G., Chemotherapy with 5-fluorouracil and folates versus chemoendocrinotherapy with 5-fluorouracil, folates and the pineal hormone melatonin in advanced gastrointestinal tract tumor patients of poor clinical status, *Arch. Geront.,* 47, 21, 1997.

39. Lissoni, P., Meregalli, S., Nosetto, L., Barni, S., Tancini, G., Fossati, V., and Maestroni, G.J.M., Increased survival time in brain glioblastomas by a radioneuroendocrine strategy with radiotherapy plus melatonin compared to radiotherapy alone, *Oncology,* 53, 43, 1996.

40. Lissoni, P., Pittalis, S., Ardizzoia, A., Brivio, F., Barni, S., Tancini, G., Pellizzoni, F., Maestroni, G.J.M., Zubelewicz, B., and Braczkowski, R., Prevention of cytokine-induced hypotension in cancer patients by the pineal hormone melatonin, *Supp. Care Cancer,* 4, 313, 1996.

41. Viviani, S., Negretti, E., Orazi, A., Sozzi, G., Santoro, A., Lissoni, P., Esposti, G., and Fraschini, F., Preliminary studies on melatonin in the treatment of myelodyspastic syndromes following cancer chemotherapy, *J. Pineal Res.,* 8, 347, 1990.

42. Brzezinski, A., Melatonin in humans, *N. Engl. J. Med.,* 336, 186, 1997.

Chapter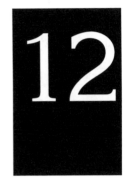

Melatonin and Reproduction

*David Solkoff, Paula Inserra,
and Ronald R. Watson*

Contents

Melatonin and Seasonal Breeders

The role of melatonin as a transmitter of photoperiodic information to the reproductive systems of animals is well known. Modification of the time span of nocturnal melatonin production constitutes the signal through which melatonin influences the reproductive axis of seasonal breeders. The pineal gland can discern the one reliable indicator of the time of year: how many hours there are between dusk and dawn. Nocturnal melatonin production increases during the long winter nights and is curtailed in the spring and summer when there are more hours of daylight. During these long winter nights, the increased production of melatonin is believed to cause reduced production of the animals' reproductive hormones which ultimately affects mating. This can be demonstrated in hamsters, whose testes atrophy and whose mating is inhibited during winter.[1]

0-8493-8564-4/99/$0.00+$.50
© 1999 by CRC Press LLC

Nature, therefore, ensures that seasonal breeders such as the Syrian hamster are born in late spring, a time of mild weather and adequate food supply. Melatonin acts on the testes of these animals to cause them to shrivel, deactivating them, thus male hamsters will not have sexual desires during the fall and winter. However, pinealectomized hamster testes failed to atrophy during winter hibernation. Without melatonin, these animals could reproduce during periods of severe weather and famine. Many of the young that would be born in the middle of winter would die, and the species as a whole could be threatened.[1] The exact role of melatonin is therefore very complex and not entirely understood.

Male hamsters maintained under natural photoperiod experience involution of the testes during the short days of winter and have normally functioning reproductive organs during the long days of spring and summer.[2] In male hamsters, reproductive inhibition is characterized by a reduction in testosterone, leuteinizing hormone (LH), follicle-stimulating hormone (FSH), and prolactin (PRL) levels. When these hormones are present in sufficient quantities, they act in concert to stimulate testes growth.[3]

A similar relationship exists in female hamsters. In short days, estrous cycles are interrupted and uteri become infantile. Not only do the ovaries fail to involute, but they also enlarge as a consequence of interstitial tissue proliferation.[4-6]

The cessation of reproductive activity in both male and female Syrian hamsters occurs when the day lengths eventually fall below the critical 12.5 hr of light daily required to maintain the neuroendocrine axis in a functionally mature state.[3,7-12] The reproductive axis remains in the dormant state throughout winter and becomes active again in spring. This dormancy is dependent on a short photoperiod and can be reversed by exposure of the animal to a long photoperiod.[3] The photoperiodic signal is transmitted to the reproductive axis of the Syrian hamster through modification of the pineal secretion of melatonin, and a decrease in photoperiod increases the nocturnal secretion of melatonin.[13-16] Pinealectomy abolishes, and the appropriate dosage of melatonin reinstates, the seasonal pattern of Syrian hamster reproduction.[3,10] Seasonality of reproduction and the transmission of photoperiodic information by melatonin has been found in many other animals, including reptiles,[10,17] birds,[10,17-21] deer,[22-23] and voles.[24] It should be noted that not all seasonally breeding animals follow the pattern of the hamster. Studies of female sheep exposed to artificial photoperiods have confirmed that exposure to short days activates the reproductive axis of ewes, while exposure to long days inhibits it.[25,26]

Melatonin and Human Breeding

Although humans are not conventionally thought of as seasonal breeders, they do have remnants of a seasonal breeding cycle. In northern Finland, which is above the Arctic Circle, there is an 8-week period in the summer during which the sun never sets. During this increased period of continuous light, the rate of conception increases significantly, suggesting that these observations may be due to seasonal changes in melatonin production. Researchers found that these women had significantly lower levels in the summer months than in the winter. As in the case of seasonally breeding animals, the increased amounts of nocturnal light apparently inhibited their production of melatonin, which consequently increased fertility.[27] Similar observations have also been seen in Eskimo women living above the Arctic Circle.[28] In regard to the majority of humans who do not live above the Arctic Circle, recent studies have described a seasonality aspect to human conception for these people, as well.[29–31] South of the Arctic, seasonal rhythm of conception is apparently influenced by environmental factors, among which photoperiod and temperature are the most obvious. A lengthening of night and a 24-hr minimum temperature of approximately 12°C seem to favor higher rates of conception.[30] It is suspected that, in humans, melatonin has the ability to inhibit the reproductive axis in both men and women and plays an essential role in determining a seasonal rhythm of conception.

In humans, melatonin determines the timing of puberty.[32] Due to a prolonged arrest in gonadal function that occurs from late infancy to the onset of puberty, sexual maturation in humans, unlike most mammals, occurs many years after birth. Because melatonin has shown antigonadotrophic effects in other mammals, it is possible that it acts as a nongonadal hormone that postpones human puberty.[33] Supporting evidence for this would be the observation that elevated nocturnal melatonin secretion occurs in patients experiencing delayed puberty.[34] Therefore, a gradual and prolonged decline in its secretion may trigger pubescence. Conversely, in patients with ideopathic precocious puberty, melatonin secretion is lower than normal.[35] Further study is needed in this area to describe melatonin's effects on male reproduction accurately. Receptors for melatonin have been detected in human spermatazoa,[36] and melatonin has been shown to reduce sperm motility.[37]

Patients with pineal tumors can have normal or undetectable melatonin levels depending on whether the tumor is of parenchymal or nonparenchymal origin and on whether the pineal gland is destroyed.[38] Sexual precocity that occurs in some patients with pineal tumors may be caused by destruction of the pineal gland and lack of melatonin, which would result in a lack of inhibition on the hypothalamic-pituitary-gonadal axis.[38,39] Excessive beta-HCG secretion, as a result of a beta-HCG-secreting pineal germinoma, can inhibit LH and melatonin secretion by increasing testosterone levels.[40]

Another melatonin-related pathologic condition of the human reproductive system is hypogonadotropic hypogonadism. Melatonin levels much greater than normal have been found in patients with hypogonadotropic hypogonadism consistent with GnRH deficiency.[41,42] Patients suffering from GnRH deficiency hypogonadism are eventually able to achieve complete maturation of pituitary-gonadal function after a gradual reduction in plasma melatonin concentrations.[43] Therefore, it is likely that excessive secretion of melatonin causes hypogonadism. By contrast, patients with hypergonadotropic hypogonadism caused by Kleinfelter's syndrome (KS) show a significant decrease in serum melatonin levels. This finding was most pronounced in low-testosterone KS and is in accordance with an earlier study that showed castrated male rats synthesize melatonin in decreased amounts. The addition of testosterone restored their ability to produce melatonin at levels seen in controls.[44] Paradoxically, melatonin levels have also been shown to decrease in the presence of high testosterone levels. This provides supporting evidence for the hypothesis that sex steroid and melatonin levels are inversely related. When sex steroids are high melatonin is inhibited, and when melatonin levels are high sex steroid levels are inhibited.[35,40] The supression of melatonin levels during testosterone treatment in male patients with GnRH deficiency[43,45] lends further credence to the existence of this inverse relationship. It is suspected that gonadotropins and gonadal steroids inhibit hypersecretion of melatonin by activating specific receptors in the pineal gland. Androgen and estrogen receptors have been demonstrated in rat pinealocytes.[46] The data described above lend value to the idea of a pineal melatonin-gonadotropin-gonadal steroid feedback mechanism which operates in a more complex way than does the pituitary gonadotropin-gonadal steroids axis. This assumes that both gonadotropins and gonadal steroids can inhibit melatonin secretion. It may also be concluded that normal testosterone levels counteract the inhibitory effects of gonadotropins on melatonin secretion, as seen in normal testosterone KS patients. Researchers believe that the activation of the gonadotropin-gonadal steroid axis, opposing melatonin hypersecretion, allows for non-seasonal reproduction in humans.[47]

Melatonin and the Menstrual Cycle

In humans, spontaneous ovulation is followed by development of a functional corporea lutea which persists for as long as 6 to 15 days. If fertilization does not occur, the corporea lutea degenerates. In animals that spontaneously ovulate, circadian inputs time the endocrine modifications preceding ovulation. In humans, the LH surge has shown a circadian pattern with a maximal incidence at late night-early morning.[48-55] Indications of melatonin's antigonadal properties include a study describing how the administration of melatonin, alone or combined with progestins, induced a significant inhibition of estradiol (E_2) and LH secretion in normal cycling women;[54] however, it is believed that melatonin has the ability to stimulate LH release in order to synchronize the pre-ovulatory rise at nighttime. In one of the first reports to describe melatonin's modulatory effect on menstrual endocrine changes, evidence was provided that acute melatonin administration, in doses capable of elevating levels of the hormone for at least 8 hr, enhances LH levels. LH pulse levels also increase in amplitude during the follicular, but not the luteal, phase of the menstrual cycle.[56] Melatonin's ability to stimulate LH release may be due to a specific action of melatonin on hypothalamic receptors — by modifying neurotransmitter and prostaglandin activity involved in GnRH regulation, melatonin may enhance GnRH release.[57-61] In another recent study, melatonin showed a stimulatory effect on LH and FSH response to physiological or submaximal GnRH stimuli in women during the follicular phase of the menstrual cycle.[62] How melatonin amplifies the pituitary response to GnRH remains unclear. The presence of specific melatonin receptors on anterior pituitaries of humans supports a direct effect of melatonin on pituitary cells.[63] It should be noted the effect of melatonin is influenced by the endocrine environment of the luteal menstrual phase. The loss of effect of melatonin in the luteal phase implies either hormone-induced modifications in the number of melatonin receptors or interruptions in the mechanisms through which melatonin exerts its stimulatory effects in the follicular phase.[64,65]

In studies investigating the effects of melatonin on prolactin (PRL) pulsatile patterns in normally cycling women, it was found that melatonin administration resulted in an upward shifting of the pulsatile secretion of PRL without significant changes in its temporal pattern.[66] This finding extends previous observations of TRH-induced PRL release after melatonin intake and points to a facilitatory effect exerted by melatonin on PRL secretion in women cycling normally.[67] These studies agree with previous studies that showed melatonin administration was able to increase PRL secretion in normal women.[68]

In human ovarian cells, melatonin seems to stimulate steroid synthesis.[69–71] Melatonin stimulates progesterone but not E_2 production from preovulatory granulosa cells, enhances basal and hCG-stimulated progesterone production from cells of day 18 to 27 corpora lutea, and stimulates androstenedione synthesis from ovarian stroma.[70,71] Melatonin may be involved in favoring the progesterone rise during the preovulatory gonadotrophin surge and in maintaining progesterone production by establishing the corpora lutea.[65] Paradoxically, some studies have found that women in the luteal phase experience lower progesterone secretion at night.[72–74] Whether melatonin contributes to this inhibition has not been determined.

Melatonin and Anovulation

Elevated levels of melatonin have been implicated in anovulatory states. In functional hypothalamic amenorrhea, melatonin levels are increased in comparison to normal cycling women. In a study of women with functional hypothalamic amenorrhea, the intravenous administration of large doses of estrogen reduced nocturnal melatonin.[75] This suggests that high melatonin levels result in a situation of depleted estrogen.

In another example of how melatonin may play a role in anovulation, women with exercise-induced amenorrhea displayed elevated nocturnal melatonin levels, with raised nocturnal peak values, delayed offset, and prolonged secretion.[76] Elevation of melatonin was associated with the amenorrheic status and not with the intensity of exercise.

An elevation of melatonin has been associated with certain psychiatric disorders associated with anovulation. In anorexic women, higher nocturnal and diurnal melatonin concentrations have been reported.[77–81] Paradoxically, other studies have shown similar melatonin levels in anorexics and control women.[82–84] Evidence, however, is currently lacking that would associate a reduction of melatonin and a return to normal cycling. It is possible that the increase in circulating melatonin does not represent the cause, but rather the consequence, of some anovulatory states. This is perhaps due to a neurotransmitter imbalance or a decreased capacity for melatonin distribution and clearance.[31]

Melatonin and Contraception

Melatonin can inhibit the reproductive system of males and females. Analogs of melatonin have been made in the laboratory which inhibit the human reproductive system when given orally. These analogs may act on the hypothalamus, pituitary, or gonads to inhibit reproduction. Melatonin is already being used as a birth-control pill.[85] Beta-Oval is a hormonal contraceptive that is composed of 75 mg of melatonin plus 0.3 mg of progestogen. It is given to females as a daily pill in order to block ovulation. It is used in Europe but is still undergoing clinical trials in the U.S. It is reported to be free of the usual side effects of contraceptive pills containing estrogen.

Conclusion

Available evidence indicates that melatonin cannot be considered at this time to be 100% progonadotrophic or 100% antigondotrophic. As previously described, its action has been shown to differ among different animal species. Even within the same species, the effect of melatonin may be different depending on the length, time, and (to a lesser degree) the quantity of its secretion or administration. Evidence points to melatonin as being an "adjuster" of many endogenous biological systems, including those relevant to reproduction. Its circadian rhythm of secretion apparently creates a functional harmony among the various biochemical players involved in mammalian reproduction.

Acknowledgments

This review was stimulated by research supported by grants from Phi Beta Psi and the Wallace Genetics Foundation, Inc. Support was also obtained from The University of Arizona Department of Molecular and Cellular Biology Undergraduate Biology Research Program, funded in part by grants from the National Science Foundation and the Howard Hughes Medical Institute.

References

1. Reiter, R.J.R. and Robinson, J., *Melatonin: Your Body's Natural Wonder Drug,* Bantam Books, New York, 1995.

2. Sorrentino, Jr., S. and Reiter, R.J.R., Pineal induced alteration of estrous cycles in blinded hamsters, *Gen. Comp. Endocrinol.,* 15, 39, 1970.

3. Reiter, R.J.R., The pineal and its hormones in the control of reproduction in mammals, *Endocr. Rev.,* 1, 109, 1980.

4. Hoffman, R.A. and Reiter, R.J.R., Responses of some endocrine organs of female hamsters to pinealectomy and light, *Life Sci.*, 5, 1147, 1966.

5. Reiter, R.J.R. and Johnson, L.Y., Pineal regulation of immunoreactive luteinizing hormone and prolactin in light-deprived female hamsters, *Fertil. Steril.*, 25, 958, 1974.

6. Seegal, R.F. and Goldman, B.D., Effects of photoperiod on cyclicity and serum gonadotrophins in the Syrian hamster, *Biol. Reprod.*, 12, 233, 1975.

7. Reiter, R.J.R., Pineal melatonin: cell biology of its synthesis and of its physiological interactions, *Endocr. Rev.*, 12, 151, 1991.

8. Yie, S.M., Niles, L.P., and Younglai, E.V., Melatonin receptors on human granulosa cell membranes, *J. Clin. Endocrinol. Metab.*, 80, 5, 1995.

9. Reiter, R.J.R., The melatonin rhythm: both a clock and a calendar. *Experientia*, 49, 654, 1993.

10. Elliot, J.A. and Goldman, B.D., Seasonal reproduction: photoperiodism and biological clocks, in Adler, N.T., Ed., *Neuroendocrinology of Reproduction: Physiology and Behavior*, Plenum Press, New York, 1981, 377.

11. Alleva, J.J., The biological clock and pineal gland: how they control seasonal fertility in the golden hamster, *Pineal Res. Rev.*, 5, 95, 1987.

12. Elliot, J.A., Circadian rhythms and photoperidic time measurement in mammals, *Fed. Proc.*, 35, 2339, 1976.

13. Rollang, M.D., Panke, E.S., and Reiter, R.J.R., Pineal melatonin content in male hamsters throughout the seasonal reproductive cycle, *Proc. Soc. Exp. Biol. Med.*, 165, 330, 1980.

14. Elliot, J.A. and Tamarkin, L., Complex circadian regulation of pineal melatonin and wheel-running in Syrian hamsters, *J. Comp. Physiol.*, 174, 469, 1994.

15. Roberts, A.C., Martensz, N.D., Hastings, M.H., and Herbert, J., Changes in photoperiod alter the daily rhythms of pineal melatonin content in hypothalamic β-endorphin content and the leuteinizing hormone response to naloxone in the male Syrian hamster, *Endocrinolgy*, 114, 141, 1985.

16. Tamarkin, L., Reppert, S.M., Klein, D.C., Pratt, B.L., and Goldman, B.D., Studies on the daily pattern of pineal melatonin in the Syrian hamster, *Endocrinology*, 107, 1525, 1980.

17. Ralph, C.L., Pineal control of reproduction: nonmammalian vertebrates, *Prog. Reprod. Biol.*, 4, 30, 1978.

18. Saxena, R.N., Malhotra, L., Kant, R., and Baweja, P.K., Effect of pinealectomy and seasonal changes on pineal antigonadotrophic activity of male Indian weaver bird *Ploceus phillipinus*, *Ind. J. Exp. Biol.*, 17, 732, 1979.

19. Cockrem, J.F., Timing of seasonal breeding in birds, with particular reference to New Zealand birds, *Reprod. Fertil. Dev.*, 7, 1, 1995.

20. Cardinalli, D.P., Cuello, A.E., Tramezzani, J.H., and Rosner, J.M., Effects of pinealectomy on the testicular function of the adult male duck, *Endocrinology*, 89, 1082, 1971.

21. Rintamaki, H., Hissa, R., Balthazart, J., and Scanes, C.G., The effect of pinealectomy on plasma levels of gonadotrophins and growth hormone in the pigeon, *Columbia livia, J. Pineal Res.,* 1, 381, 1984.

22. Elorata, E., Timisjarvi, J., Nieman, M., Ojutkangas, V., Leppaluoto, V., and Vakkuri, O., Seasonal and daily patterns in melatonin secretion in female reindeer and their calves, *Endocrinology,* 130, 1645, 1992.

23. Asher, G.W., Veldhuizen, F.A., Morrow, C.J., and Duganzich, D.M., Effect of exogenous melatonin on prolactin secretion, lactogenesis, and reproductive seasonality of adult female red deer, *Cervus elaphus, J. Reprod. Fertil.,* 100, 11, 1994.

24. Farrar, G.M. and Clarke, J.R., Effect of chemical sympathectomy and pinealectomy upon gonads of voles (*Microtus agrestis*) exposed to short photoperiod, *Neuroendocrinology,* 22, 134, 1976.

25. Mauleon, P. and Rougeot, J., Regulation des saisons sexuelles chez des brebis de races differentes au moyen de divers rhythmes lumineux, *Ann. Biol. Anim. Bioch. Biophys.,* 2, 209, 1962.

26. Legan, S.J. and Karsch, F.J., Photoperiodic seasonal control of breeding in ewes: modulation of the negative feedback action of estradiol, *Biol. Reprod.,* 23, 1061, 1980.

27. Rojansky, N., Brzezinski, A., and Schenker, J.G., Seasonality in human reproduction: an update, *Human Reprod.,* 7, 735–745, 1992.

28. Cook, F.A., Medical observations among the Esquimaux, *Trans. N.Y. Obstet. Soc.,* 3, 282–291, 1894.

29. Roennerberg, T. and Aschoff, J., Annual rhythm of human reproduction. 1. Biology, sociology, or both?, *J. Biol. Rhythms,* 5, 195–216, 1990.

30. Roennerberg, T. and Aschoff, J., Annual rhythm of human reproduction. 2. Environmental correlations, *J. Biol. Rhythms,* 5, 217–239, 1990.

31. Cagnacci, A. and Volpe, A., Influence of melatonin and photoperiod on animal and human reproduction, *J. Endocrinol. Invest.,* 19, 382–411, 1996.

32. Arendt, J., Melatonin: miracle or myth? *Organons Mag. Women Health,* 3, 37–40, 1997.

33. Wurtman, R.J. and Brzezinski, A., The pineal gland: its possible roles in human reproduction, *Obstet. Gyn. Survey,* 43(4), 197–207, 1988.

34. Cohen, H.N., Hay, I.D., Annesley, T.M., Beastall, G.H., Wallace, A.M., Apooner, R., Eastwood, T.P., and Klee, G.G., Serum immunoreactive melatonin in boys with delayed puberty, *Clin. Endocrinol.,* 17, 527–531, 1982.

35. Waldhauser, F., Boepple, P.A., Schemper, M., Mansfield, M.J., and Crowley, Jr., W.F., Serum melatonin in central precocious puberty is lower than in age-matched prepubertal children, *J. Clin. Endocrinol. Metab.,* 73, 793–796, 1991.

36. van Buren, R.J., Pitout, M.J., Van Aswegen, C.H., and Theron, J.J., Putative melatonin receptor in human spermatazoa, *Clin. Biochem.,* 25, 125–127, 1992.

37. Irez, T.O., Senol, H., Alagoz, M., Basmaciogullari, C., Turan, F., Kuru, D., and Ertungelap, E., Effects of indoleamines on sperm motility *in vitro, Human Reprod.,* 7, 987–990, 1992.

38. Vorkapic, P., Waldhauser, F., Bruckner, R., Biegelmayer, C., Schmidbauer, M., and Pendl, G., Serum melatonin levels: a new neurodiagnostic tool in pineal region tumors?, *Neurosurgery*, 21, 817–824, 1987.

39. Styne, D.M., Puberty and its disorders in boys, *Endocrinol. Metab. Clin. N. Am.*, 20, 43–69, 1991.

40. Luboshitsky, R., Tiosano,D., Ben-Harush, M., Thuma, I., Ayash, A., Lavie, P., and Etzioni, A., Pseudo-precocious puberty in a male patient and the melatonin-testosterone relationship, *J. Ped. Endocrinol. Metab.*, 8, 295–299, 1995.

41. Brzezinski, A., Lynch, H.J., Seibel, M.M., Deng, M.H., Nader, T.M., and Wurtman, R.J., The circadian rhythm of plasma melatonin during the normal menstrual cycle and in amenorrheic women, *J. Clin. Endocrinol. Metab.*, 66, 891–895, 1988.

42. Berga, S.L., Mortola, J.F., and Yen, S.S.C., Amplification of nocturnal melatonin secretion in women with functional hypothalamic amenorrhea, *J. Clin. Endocrinol. Metab.*, 66, 242–244, 1988.

43. Puig-Domingo, M., Webb, S.M., Serrano, J., Peinado, M.A., Corcoy, R., Ruscalleda, J., Reiter, R.J., and De Leiva, A., Brief report: melatonin-related hypogonadotropic hypogonadism, *New Engl. J. Med.*, 5, 1356–1359, 1992.

44. Daya, S. and Potgeiter, B., The effect of castration, testosterone, and estradiol on ^{14}C-serontin metabolism by organ cultures of male rat pineal glands, *Experientia*, 41, 275–276, 1985.

45. Luboshitsky, R., Lavi, S., Thuma, I., and Lavie, P., Testosterone treatment alters melatnin concentrations in male patients with GnRH deficiency, *J. Clin. Endocrinol. Metab.*, 81, 770-774, 1996.

46. Ciocca, D.R. and Vargas-Roig, L.M., Estrogen receptors in human nontarget tissues: biological and clinical implications, *Endocrine Rev.*, 16, 35–62, 1995.

47. Luboshitsky, R., Wagner, O., Lavi, S., Herer, P., and Lavie, P. Abnormal melatonin secretion in male patients with hypogonadism. *J. Mol. Neurosci.*, 7, 91–98, 1996.

48. Zimmermann, R.C., Schroder, S., Baars, S., Schumacher, M., and Weise, H.C., Melatonin and the ovulatory luteinizing hormone surge, *Fertil. Steril.*, 54, 612, 1990.

49. Kapen, S., Boyer, R., Hellman, L., and Weitzman, E.D., Episodic release of luteinizing hormone at mid-menstrual cycle in normal adult women, *J. Clin. Endocrinol. Metab.*, 36, 724, 1973.

50. Edwards, R.G., Steptoe, P.C., and Purdy, J.M., Establishing full-term human pregnancies using cleaving embryos grown *in vitro*, *Br. J. Obstet. Gynecol.*, 87, 737, 1980.

51. Edwards, R.G., Test-tube babies, *Nature*, 293, 253, 1981.

52. Testart, J., Frydman, R., and Roger, M., Seasonal influence of diurnal rhythms in the onset of the plasma luteinizing hormone surge in women, *J. Clin. Endocrinol. Metab.*, 55, 374, 1982.

53. Brzezinski, A., Lynch, H.L., Wurtman, R.J., and Seibel, M.M., Possible contribution of melatonin to the timing of the luteinizing hormone surge, *New Engl. J. Med.*, 316, 1550, 1987.

54. Voordouw, B.G., Euser, R., Verdonk, R.E., Alberda, B.T., De Jong, F.H., Drogendijk, A.C., Fauser, B.C., and Cohen, M., Melatonin and melatonin-progestin combinations: a pituitary-ovarian function in women and can inhibit ovulation, *J. Clin. Endocrinol. Metab.*, 74, 108–117, 1992.

55. Rossmanith, W. and Yen, S.S.C., Sleep-associated decrease in LH-pulse frequency during the early follicular phase of the menstrual cycle: evidence for an opiodergic mechanism, *J. Clin. Endocrinol. Metab.*, 65, 713, 1987.

56. Cagnacci, A., Soldani, R., and Yen, S.S.C., Exogenous melatonin enhances luteinizing hormone levels of women in the follicular but not in the luteal menstrual phase, *Fertil. Steril.*, 63:5, 996-999, 1995.

57. Morgan, P.J. and Williams, L.M., Central melatonin receptors: implication for a mode of action, *Experientia*, 45, 955–965, 1989.

58. Glass, J.D., Neuroendocrine regulation of seasonal reproduction by the pineal gland and melatonin, *Pineal Res. Rev.*, 6, 219–259, 1988.

59. Kao, L.W. and Weisz, J., Release of gonadotropin releasing hormone (GnRH) from isolated perifused medial-basal hypothalamus by melatonin, *Endocrinology* 100, 1723–1726, 1977.

60. Richardson, S.B., Prasad, J.A., and Hollander, C.S., Acetylcholine, melatonin, and potassium depolarization stimulate release of luteinizing hormone-releasing hormone (LHRH) from rat hypothalamus *in vitro, Proc. Natl. Acad. Sci. USA*, 79, 2686–2689, 1982.

61. Rasmussen, D.D., Diurnal modulation of rat hypothalamic gonadotropin releasing hormone (GRH) release by melatonin *in vitro, J. Endocrinol. Invest.*, 16, 1–7, 1993.

62. Cagnacci, A., Paoletti, A.M., Soldani, R., Orru, M., Maschio, E., and Melis, G.B., Melatonin enhances the luteinizing hormone (LH) and follicle stimulating hormone (FSH) responses to gonadotropin releasing hormone (GRH) in the follicular, but not in the luteal, menstrual phase, *J. Clin. Endocrinol. Metab.*, 80(4), 1095–1099, 1995.

63. Weaver, D.R., Stehle, J.H., Stopa, E.G., and Reppert, S.M., Melatonin receptors in human hypothalamus and pituitary: implications for circadian and reproductive responses to melatonin, *J. Clin. Endocrinol. Metab.*, 76, 295–301, 1993.

64. Seltzer, A., Viswanathan, M., and Saavedra, J.M., Melatonin-binding sites in brain and caudal arteries of the female rat during the estrus cycle and after estrogen administration, *Endocrinology*, 130, 1896–1902, 1992.

65. Yen, S.S.C., The human menstrual cycle: neuroendocrine regulation, in Yen, S.S.C. and Jaffe, R.B., Eds., *Reproductive Endocrinology*, 3rd ed., Saunders, Philadelphia, 1991, 273–308.

66. Terzolo, M., Revelli, A., Guidetti, D., Piovesan, A., Cassoni, P., Paccotti, P., Angeli, A., and Massobrio, M., Evening administration of melatonin enhances the pulsatile secretion of prolactin but not of LH and TSH in normally cycling women, *Clin. Endocrinol.*, 39, 185–191, 1993.

67. Terzolo, M., Piovesan, A., Osella, G., Torta, M., Buniva, T., Paccotti, P., Wierdis, T., and Angeli, A., Exogenous melatonin enhances the TRH-induced prolactin release in normally cycling women, a sex-specfic effect, *Gynecol. Endocrinol.*, 5, 83–94, 1991.

68. Bispink, G., Zimmermann, R., Weise, H.C., and Leidenberger, F., Influence of melatonin on the sleep-independent component of prolactin secretion, *J. Pineal Res.,* 8, 97–106, 1990.

69. Yie, S.M., Brown, G.M., Liu, G.Y., Collins, J.A., Daya, S., Hughes, E.G., Foster, W.G., and Younglai, E.V., Melatonin and steroids in human preovulatory follicular fluid: seasonal variation and granulosa cell steroid production, *Human Reprod.,* 10, 50, 1995.

70. Webley, G.E. and Luck, M.R., Melatonin directly stimulates the secretion of proges-terone by human and bovine granulosa cells *in vitro, J. Reprod. Fertil.,* 78, 711, 1986.

71. MacPhee, A.A., Cole, F.E., and Rice, B.F., The effect of melatonin on steroidogenesis by the human ovary *in vitro, J. Clin. Endocrinol. Metab.,* 40, 688, 1975.

72. Spies, H.G., Mahoney, C.J., Norman, R.L., Clifton, D.K., and Resko, J.A., Evidence for a diurnal rhythm in ovarian steroid secretion in the Rhesus monkey, *J. Clin. Endocrinol. Metab.,* 39, 347, 1974.

73. Veldhuis, J.D., Christiansen, E., Evans, W.S., Kolp, L.A., Rogol, A.D., and Johnson, M.L., Physiological profiles of episodic progesterone release during the midluteal phase of the human menstrual cycle: analysis of circadian and ultradian rhythms, discrete pulse properties, and correlations with simultaneous luteinizing hormone release, *J. Clin. Endocrinol. Metab.,* 66, 414, 1988.

74. Rossmanith, W.G., Laughlin, G.A., Mortola, J.F., Johnson, Veldhuis, J.D., and Yen, S.S.C., Pulsatile co-secretion of estradiol and progesterone by the midluteal phase corpus luteum: temporal link to luteinizing hormone pulses, *J. Clin. Endocrinol. Metab.,* 70, 990, 1990.

75. Okatani, Y. and Sagara, Y., Enhanced nocturnal melatonin secretion in women with functional secondary amenorrhea: relationship to opioid system and endogenous estrogen levels, *Hormone Res.,* 43, 194, 1995.

76. Laughlin, G.A., Loucks, A.B., and Yen, S.S.C., Marked augmentation of nocturnal melatonin secretion in amenorrheic athletes, but not cycling athletes: unaltered by opiodergic or dopaminergic blockade, *J. Clin. Endocrinol. Metab.,* 73, 1321, 1991.

77. Tortosa, F., Puig-Domingo, M., Peinado, M.A., Oriola, J., Webb S.M., and de Leiva, A., Enhanced circadian rhythm of melatonin in anorexia nervosa, *Acta Endocrinol. (Copenhagen)*, 120, 584, 1989.

78. Brambilla, F., Fraschini, F., Espositi, G., Bossolo, P.A., Marelli, G., and Ferrari, E., Melatonin circadian rhythm in anorexia nervosa and obesity, *Psychiatr. Res.,* 23, 267, 1988.

79. Ferrari, E., Poppa, S., Bossolo, P.A., Comis, S., Espositi, G., Licini, V., Fraschini, F., and Brambilla, F., Melatonin and pituitary-gonadal function in disorders of eating behavior, *J. Pineal Res.,* 7, 115, 1989.

80. Arendt, J., Bhanji, S., Franey, C., and Mattingly, D., Plasma melatonin levels in anorexia nervosa. *Br. J. Psychiatry* 161, 361, 1992.

81. Bearn, J., Treasure, J., Murphy, M., Franey, C., Arendt, J., Wheeler, M., and Checkley, S.A., A study of sulphatoxymelatonin excretion and gonadotrophin status during weight gain in anorexia nervosa, *Br. J. Psychiatry,* 152, 372, 1988.

82.   Kennedy, S.H., Brown, G.M., Garfinkel, P.E., McVey, G., Costa, D., and Parienti, V.,
       Sulphatoxymelatonin: an index of depression in anorexia nervosa and bulimia nervosa,
       Psychiatry Res., 32, 221, 1990.

83.   Kennedy, S.H., Brown, G.M., Ford, C.G., and Ralevski, E., The acute effects of
       starvation on 6-sulphatoxymelatonin output in subgroups of patients with anorexia
       nervosa, *Psychneuroendocrinology,* 18, 131, 1993.

84.   Mortola, J.F., Laughlin, G.A., and Yen, S.S.C., Melatonin rhythms in women with
       anorexia nervosa and bulimia nervosa, *J. Clin. Endocrinol. Metab.,* 77, 1540, 1993.

85.   Jones, R.E., *Human Reproductive Biology,* 2nd ed., Academic Press, San Diego,
       1997, 284.

Chapter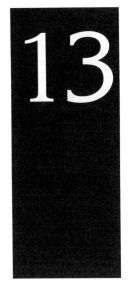

Alzheimer's Disease and Melatonin: Functional and Pathological Considerations

Charles P. Maurizi

Contents

0-8493-8564-4/99/$0.00+$.50
© 1999 by CRC Press LLC

Introduction

Alzheimer's disease is a progressive degenerative central nervous system disease with the loss of memory for recent events as a common presenting sign. Symptoms of depression are common early in the disease. Mild personality changes occur with apathy and quiet withdrawal from social interactions. In the middle stages, individual may be querulous, slovenly, irritable, or agitated. Late in the disease, patients may be bedridden, mute, inattentive, and uncooperative.

The prevalence of Alzheimer's disease increases with age. It is estimated that the percentage of the population affected doubles during every decade after age 65, with a 10% prevalence in those over 65, 20% in those over 75, and 40% in those greater than 85 years of age.[1] Patients dying with severe Alzheimer's disease have global atrophy of the frontal, parietal, and temporal lobes of the brain; however, demonstrable histological loss of neurons is regional and laminar and not global.[2] Brain areas that have significant neuron depletion include the hippocampus, the entorhinal cortex, the locus coeruleus, and the dorsal raphe nucleus.

Pineal gland secretion of melatonin significantly decreases with increasing age. When compared to age-matched controls, an even more profound decrease of melatonin production occurs in Alzheimer's disease.[3-5] Unconventional concepts can link the functional and neuropathological findings in Alzheimer's disease to the deficiency of melatonin.

Unconventional Useful Concepts

Melatonin, Vasotocin, and REM Sleep

Sleep induction by melatonin was observed 30 years ago.[6] In a series of experiments, the endocrinologist Stephan Pavel has demonstrated a role for melatonin in rapid eye movement (REM) sleep. Melatonin is a releasing factor for the nonapeptide vasotocin. Vasotocin, the apparent phylogenetic precursor of oxytocin and vasopressin, is released into the cerebrospinal fluid (CSF) with a circadian sensitivity to melatonin.[7] Extremely small amounts of vasotocin in the ventricular system can have systemic effects.[8] In human beings, vasotocin is present in the CSF during REM sleep and not at other times.[9] REM sleep is associated with vivid and sometimes bizarre dreams. Pavel induced REM sleep with the intranasal application of vasotocin.[10] REM sleep aids in memory formation and the resolution of emotion.[11-13] States with deficient melatonin production could be associated with abnormal sleep, impaired affect, and inadequate memory.

Cerebrospinal Fluid Circulation

The currently held theory of absorption of CSF through the arachnoid granule-superior sagittal sinus system is based on infusion experiments in cadavers and on

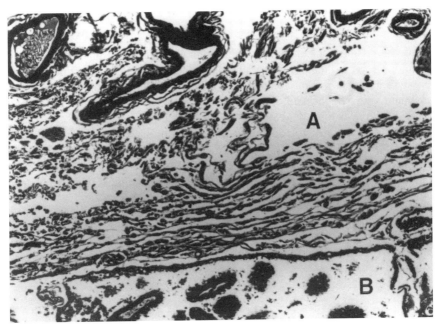

FIGURE 1
Portal to the lateral ventricle (H&E stain, original magnification 100×). **(A)** CSF in choroid fissure. **(B)** CSF in the lateral ventricle. Between A and B is the tela choroidae composed of a loose pial membrane covered by ependyma on the ventricular surface. (For additional microphotographs of ventricular portals, see Reference 38.)

infusion experiments at lethal pressure in animals.[14] What the experiments demonstrate is the site of forceful rupture of the membranes covering the central nervous system and not a physiological process.

The arachnoid granule-superior sagittal sinus theory of CSF resorption fails to explain the behavior of substances circulating in the CSF. The pattern of deposition of corpora amylacea on the surface of the brain suggests that after exiting the ventricular system, CSF transits the basilar cisternae to the tela choroidae of the choroid plexuses for re-entry into the ventricular system.[15] Radiographic studies in communicating hydrocephalus and magnetic resonance imaging (MRI) findings in superficial siderosis provide observations that are impossible to explain with the currently held theory of CSF circulation.[16]

Superficial siderosis and experimental superficial siderosis demonstrate brain damage caused by toxic "free" iron within the CSF. Patterns of damage clearly demonstrate the physiological circulation of CSF with carriage of fluid to and through the tela choroidae. The tela choroidae is composed of a loose pial membrane and an ependymal lining. This tissue is a portal for CSF re-entry into the ventricular system (see Figure 1).

The Erasable Scratch Pad

An entorhinal-hippocampal complex is the neural site for the temporary storage of new information and the storage area for dream subjects.[17] Electrical stimulation of the entorhinal-hippocampal complex can elicit dream-like memories;[18] however, these memories are ephemeral. It has been known for decades that bilateral destruction of the hippocampus destroys the ability to form new memory. Patients with bilateral hippocampal destruction have dreams that are described as short, simple, repetitious, stereotyped, and lacking emotional impact.[19] Sleep has a role in the function of the scratch pad. We have all experienced an interesting dream, which we intend to share with others, but after further sleep and upon awakening the content of the dream is lost. The scratch pad has been erased.

Alzheimer's Disease and Melatonin

Alzheimer's Disease and Sleep

Using the described unconventional concepts, evidence supporting a profound and prolonged deficiency of melatonin in ventricular CSF as the cause of the functional and pathological findings in Alzheimer's disease will be presented. While memory loss is widely recognized as a hallmark of Alzheimer's disease, disturbed sleep is also present early in the disease. Abnormal sleep patterns are predictive of later intellectual failure compared to those with normal sleep.[20] Aged normal subjects have less stage 3 sleep, stage 4 sleep, and REM sleep and more wakefulness than do normal young adults. Compared with aged normal subjects, patients with Alzheimer's disease have even less stage 3 sleep, no stage 4 sleep, very little REM sleep, and more frequent awakenings.[21] The quality of sleep continues to deteriorate as the disease progresses.

Demented patients have disturbance of the sleep/wake cycle with increasing daytime naps and less sleep at night. They also frequently have "sundown syndrome" with confusion, agitation, and delirium during the evening or at night.[22-24] The "sundown syndrome" and nighttime wakefulness in demented patients are serious difficulties for caregivers to contend with in the home.

Abnormalities of sleep noted in normal aging and in Alzheimer's disease parallel the decreased production of melatonin. In elderly patients, insomnia is directly correlated to insufficient melatonin.[25] Exogenous administration of melatonin improves the quality of sleep in aged subjects.[26-28] Such treatment corrects sleep/wake rhythms in blind and melatonin-deficient individuals.[29,30] Melatonin therapy should improve sleep and the sleep/wake cycle in patients with early Alzheimer's disease.

Melatonin and Cerebrospinal Fluid

Nighttime levels of melatonin in the CSF of the lateral ventricles are five to ten times greater than simultaneously sampled blood in goats, sheep and calves.[31-33] Similar experimental observations have not been confirmed in normal human beings for obvious reasons. High concentrations of melatonin in the ventricular CSF can be explained by release of melatonin directly into the surrounding CSF, which then transits the choroid fissure and then passes through the tela choroidae into the lateral ventricle (see Figures 2 and 3).

Melatonin is a lipophilic substance with unique antioxidant characteristics. It quenches the highly reactive hydroxyl radical, with suicidal modification of the chemical structure of melatonin. In addition, the neurohormone limits the production of oxygen radicals by inhibiting monoamine oxidase, cyclo-oxygenase, nitric oxide synthase, and a gene for lipooxygenase.[34–37]

A hypothesis has been proposed that links the loss of ventricular fluid CSF melatonin with the pattern of neuron loss in Alzheimer's disease.[38] Because melatonin is lipophilic, it can pass through cell membranes. Skin patches can deliver systemic melatonin. Brain tissue in close contact with the ventricular CSF would be in a privileged position for high intracellular melatonin levels, with elevated antioxidant protection compared to other tissue. For instance, as CSF enters the lateral ventricle, the melatonin-enriched fluid bathes the ependyma covering the alveus of the hippocampus. The alveus contains fibers from the CA1 area of the hippocampus and some fibers from the entorhinal cortex. These tissues have selective cell loss and early histologic change in Alzheimer's disease and are part of the erasable scratch pad.

Vulnerability of the Erasable Scratch Pad

The brain accounts for 2% of body weight while consuming 20% of the oxygen, making the nervous system the "most oxidative" tissue of the body.[39] The CA1 area of the hippocampus is more sensitive to both oxygen and glucose deprivation than the brain in general. During such deprivations, extensive cellular destruction can occur in the CA1 area, while other neural tissue is spared. This suggests a greater need for and utilization of these metabolites. The erasable scratch pad may be the "most oxidative" tissue in the brain. The "most oxidative" component of a cell is mitochondrial oxidative phosphorylation, which is stated to consume more than 90% of cellular oxygen.[40] Thus, the mitochondria in the erasable scratch pad may be the "most oxidative" elements of the "most oxidative" area of the "most oxidative" tissue in the body. Teleologically, brain tissue meeting the metabolic needs of chemical and structural plasticity for new memory formation would require vigorous consumption of energy. Is there evidence that a melatonin deficiency could cause the destruction present in the entorhinal-hippocampal complex present in Alzheimer's disease?

A Scenario

Loss of intracellular melatonin level, with inadequate suppression of oxygen radical generating systems, increases the substrate available for the generation of the damaging hydroxyl radical. At the same time, melatonin is not available to quench the radicals that are produced. Hydroxyl radicals would then be free to react, with great

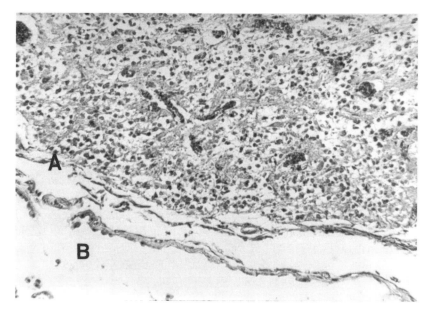

FIGURE 2
Pineal gland (H&E stain, original magnification 100×). **(A)** Surface of the pineal gland. **(B)** CSF of the basal cistern.

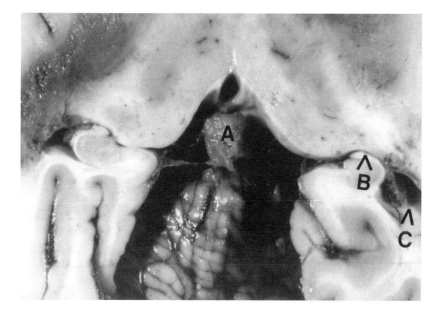

FIGURE 3
Inferior surface of a horizontal section of the brain just superior to the pineal gland. **(A)** Pineal gland, **(B)** choroid fissure, **(C)** lateral ventricle. (Note that the pineal gland is separated from the lateral ventricle only by the meager capsule of the pineal gland and the tela choroidae.[2])

speed, with almost every molecule found in living cells, including DNA, proteins, membrane lipids, and carbohydrates.[40] With a deficient antioxidant system, hydroxyl radicals generated by mitochondrial metabolism damage nearby structures.

The erasable scratch pad normally has enhanced intracellular melatonin, because of its anatomic relationship to the tela choroidae of the lateral ventricle. Therefore, the absolute decrease of melatonin levels intracellularly in the entorhinal-hippocampal complex would be even greater than the marked deficiency found in the serum of patients with Alzheimer's disease. In addition, neurons have a high ratio of surface area to volume due to the cellular elongations of axons and dendrites, and they have membranes that are rich in polyunsaturated fatty acid side chains which are especially sensitive to radical attack.[41,42]

Evidence Supporting the Scenario

Brain tissue from patients dying of Alzheimer's disease has increased formation of radicals, when compared to brain tissue from controls.[41] Clear evidence of oxidative stress in Alzheimer's disease is found in proteins, carbohydrates, mitochondrial DNA, mitochondrial cytochrome c oxidase, mitochondrial alpha-ketoglutarate dehydrogenase, and with the induction of heat shock proteins.[29,43–49] Finding damaged mitochondrial structures seems logical because of proximity to the flame of hydroxyl radical generation. With significant mitochondrial damage, oxidative phosphorylation could become uncoupled and even more radicals formed. ALZ-50 is an antigen found in brain tissue from patients with Alzheimer's disease. The expression of ALZ-50 can be induced by chemically uncoupling oxidative phosphorylation.[50]

Oxidative stress is one of the mechanisms that induces apoptosis.[51] Active apoptotic cell death is found in the hippocampus of patients dying of Alzheimer's disease.[52] Melatonin has been shown to protect neurons from apoptosis caused by oxidative stress.[53] Although cell death is regional and laminar in Alzheimer's disease, there is global atrophy of the frontal, parietal, and temporal lobes of the brain. With sufficient damage to the erasable scratch pad, new memory is not formed while awake or during REM sleep. Without the stimulus of new memory, the neocortex undergoes disuse atrophy.

Identification of Melatonin Deficiencies

If deficient melatonin is the cause of Alzheimer's disease, then early identification of individuals at risk is important. Nighttime collection of serum for quantitation of melatonin levels is simple but inconvenient. Collection of an overnight urine sample for the quantitation of melatonin metabolites is more convenient for the patient but subject to errors in collection and handling. A potential method of Alzheimer's disease patient identification would entail a device to record overnight temperature. Melatonin plays a significant role in the suppression of nighttime temperature in human beings.[54,55] Individuals who do not lower temperature in a normal fashion could undergo further testing to document a melatonin deficiency.

Melatonin Therapy

The etiology of a pineal gland failure in demented patients is unknown. A pharmacological agent that stimulates the production of melatonin in normal people and various central nervous system disorders fails to increase the production of the substance in demented patients.[56,57] This is an indication that exogenous melatonin will be needed for treatment.

In a recent review, the use of melatonin has been shown to be safe in human beings;[58] however, the most effective dose and manner of treatment are unknown. Until more information becomes available, it seems prudent to recommend the smallest dose that corrects the sleep disorder and normalizes overnight body temperature. A dose of 1 to 2 mg given orally has been effective for sleep improvement in elderly subjects.

Ultimately, emulation of normal intraventricular CSF levels and rhythms of melatonin might be desirable. Recycling of CSF through the ventricular system has been suggested to pace ultradian rhythms, such as REM sleep.[15] If ventricular CSF levels of melatonin are pulsatile, the ideal therapy may require a matching rhythm.

Conclusion

An understanding of the neuropathology of Alzheimer's disease requires abandonment of the effete arachnoid granule-superior sagittal sinus theory of CSF absorption. In superficial siderosis, "free" iron is a toxic substance that catalyzes the generation of hydroxyl radicals, and the flow of CSF through the ventricular system, the basilar cisternae, and the tela choroidae demarcates tissue damage. In Alzheimer's disease, the distribution of cellular damage is more subtle. Normally active neural tissue in contact with ventricular CSF is protected by high levels of melatonin. With the loss of melatonin's hydroxyl radical quenching ability, the brain becomes a victim of its own metabolism. The most active tissue of the brain is the most vulnerable.

Microscopic features of Alzheimer's disease include neurofibrillary tangles, senile plaques, granulo-vacuolar degeneration, amyloid angiopathy, apoptosis, and pigment incontinence. All of these features may prove to be ashes caused by the flame of the hydroxyl radical.

The cause of decreased production of melatonin in aging and Alzheimer's disease is unknown. Earliest clinical signs of the deficiency are related to malfunction of the entorhinal-hippocampal complex. Disturbed memory and abnormal sleep herald the onset of disease. It is hoped that these signs will prove to be functional and reversible with adequate melatonin therapy. The optimal treatment regimen should be sought. Delay in identification and treatment may lead to irreversible cellular damage.

References

1. Khachaturian, Z.S. and Rabebaugh, T.S., *Alzheimer's Disease. Cause(s), Diagnosis, Treatment and Care,* CRC Press, Boca Raton, FL, 1996, 3.

2. Hyman, B.T. and Gomez-Isla, T., Alzheimer's disease is a laminar, regional, and neural system specific disease, not a global brain disease, *Neurobiol. Aging,* 15, 353, 1994.

3. Mishima, K., Okawa, M., Hishikawa, Y., Hozumi, S., Hori, H., and Takahashi, K., Morning bright light therapy for sleep and behavior disorders in elderly patients with dementia, *Acta Psychiatr. Scand.,* 89, 1, 1994.

4. Nair, N.P.V., Hariharasubramanian, N., Pilapil, C., and Thavumday, J.X., Plasma melatonin rhythm in normal aging and Alzheimer's disease, *J. Neural Trans.,* 21(suppl.), 494, 1986.

5. Skene, D.J., Vivien-Roels, B., Sparks, D.L., Hunsaker, D.L., Pévet, P., Ravid, D., and Swabb, D.F., Daily variation in the concentration of melatonin and 5-methoxytryptohol in the human pineal gland: effect of age and Alzheimer's disease, *Brain Res.,* 528, 170, 1990.

6. Barkas, J., DaCosta, F., and Spector, S., Acute pharmacology of melatonin, *Nature,* 214, 919, 1967.

7. Pavel, S. and Goldstein, R., Further evidence that melatonin represents the releasing hormone for pineal vasotocin, *J. Endocrinol.,* 82, 1, 1979.

8. Pavel, S., Cristoveanu, A., Goldstein, R., and Calb, M., Inhibition of release of corticotropin releasing hormone in cats by extremely small amounts of vasotocin injected into the third ventricle of the brain. Evidence for the involvement of 5-hydroxytryptamine-containing neurons, *Endocrinology,* 101, 672, 1977.

9. Pavel, S., Goldstein, R., Popviciu, L., Corfariu, O., and Foldes, A., and Farkas, E., Pineal vasotocin: REM sleep-dependent release into cerebrospinal fluid of man, *Waking Sleeping,* 3, 347, 1979.

10. Pavel, S., Goldstein, R., Petrescu, M., and Popa, M., REM sleep induction in prepubertal boys by vasotocin, *Peptides,* 2, 245, 1981.

11. Greenberg, R., Pillard, R., and Pearlman, C., The effect of dream (stage REM) deprivation on adaption to stress, *Psychosom. Med.,* 34, 257, 1972.

12. Greenberg, R., Pearlman, C., Schwartz, W.R., and Grossman, H.Y., Memory, emotion, and REM sleep, *J. Abnormal Psychol.,* 92, 378, 1983.

13. Scrima L., Isolated REM sleep facilitates recall of complex associative information, *Psychophysiology,* 19, 252, 1982.

14. Maurizi, C.P., Recirculation of cerebrospinal fluid through the tela choroidae is why high levels of melatonin can be found in the lateral ventricles, *Med. Hypotheses,* 35, 154, 1991.

15. Maurizi, C.P., The circulation and function of cerebrospinal fluid, *Med. Hypotheses,* 15, 155, 1984.

16. Maurizi, C.P., Superficial siderosis of the brain: roles for CSF circulation, iron and the hydroxyl radical, *Med. Hypotheses,* 47, 261, 1996.

17. Maurizi, C.P., The function of dreams (REM sleep): roles for the hippocampus, melatonin, monoamines and vasotocin, *Med. Hypotheses,* 23, 433, 1987.

18. Halgren, E., Walter, R.D., Cherlow, D.G., and Grandell, P.H., Mental phenomena evoked by electrical stimulation of the hippocampal formation and amygdala, *Brain*, 101, 83, 1978.

19. Torda, C., Dreams of subjects with bilateral hippocampal lesions, *Acta Psychiat. Scand.*, 45, 277, 1969.

20. Prinz P.N., Sleep patterns in the healthy aged: interrelationships with intellectual function, *J. Gerontol.*, 32, 179, 1977.

21. Prinz, P.N., Peskind, E.R., Vitaliano, P.P., Raskind, M.A., Eisdorfer, C., Zemuznikov, N., and Gerber, C.J., Changes in the sleep and waking EEGs of nondemented and demented elderly subjects, *J. Am. Geriatr. Soc.*, 30, 86, 1982.

22. Vitiello, M.V. Bliwise, D.L., and Prinz, P.N., Sleep in Alzheimer's disease and the sundown syndrome, *Neurology*, 42(suppl. 6), 83, 1992.

23. Little, J.T., Satlin, A., Sunderland, T., and Volicer, L., Sundown syndrome in severely demented patients with probable Alzheimer's disease, *J. Geriatr. Psychiatry Neurol.*, 8, 103, 1995.

24. Bliwise, D.L., Yesavage, J.A., and Tinklenberg, J.R., Sundowning and rate of decline in mental function in Alzheimer's disease, *Dementia*, 3, 335, 1992.

25. Haimov, I., Laudon, M., Zisapel, N., Souroujon, M., Nof, D., Shlitner, A., Herer, P., Tzischinsky, O., and Lavie, P., Sleep disorders and melatonin rhythms in elderly people, *Br. Med. J.*, 309, 167, 1994.

26. Haimov, I., Lavie, P., Laudon, M., Herer, P., Vigder, C., and Zisapel, N., Melatonin replacement therapy of elderly insomniacs, *Sleep*, 18, 498, 1995.

27. Garfinkel, D., Laudon, M., and Zisapel, N., Improvement of sleep quality in elderly people by controlled-release melatonin, *Lancet*, 346, 541, 1995.

28. Wurtman, R.J. and Zhdanova, I., Improvement in sleep quality by melatonin, *Lancet*, 346, 1491, 1995.

29. Palm, L., Blennow, G., and Wetterberg, L., Correction of non-24-hour sleep/wake cycle by melatonin in a blind retarded boy, *Ann. Neurol.*, 29, 336, 1991.

30. Petterborg, L.J., Thalen, B.E., Kjellman, B.F., and Wetterberg, L., Effect of melatonin replacement on serum hormone rhythms in a patient lacking endogenous melatonin, *Brain Res. Bull.*, 27, 181, 1991.

31. Kanematsu, N., Mori, Y., Hayashi, S., and Hoshino, K., Presence of a distinct 24-hour melatonin rhythm in the ventricular cerebrospinal fluid of the goat, *J. Pineal Res.*, 7, 143, 1989.

32. Shaw, P.F., Kennaway, D.J., and Seamark, R.F., Evidence of high concentrations of melatonin in the lateral ventricular cerebrospinal fluid of sheep, *J. Pineal Res.*, 6, 201, 1989.

33. Hedland, L., Lischko, M.M., Rollag, M.D., and Niswender, G.D., Melatonin: daily cycle in plasma and cerebrospinal fluid of calves, *Science*, 195, 686, 1977.

34. Urry, R.L. and Ellis, L.C., Monoamine oxidase activity of the hypothalamus and pituitary, changes in photoperiod of additions of melatonin *in vitro*, *Experientia*, 31, 891, 1975.

35. Reiter, R.J., Pablos, M.I., Agapito, T.T., and Guerrero, J.M., Melatonin in the context of the free radical theory of aging, *Ann. N.Y. Acad. Sci.,* 786, 362, 1996.

36. Franchi, A.M., Gimeno, M.F., Cardinali, D.P., and Vacas, M.I., Melatonin, 5-methoxytryptamine and some of their analogs as cyclo-oxygenase inhibitors in rat medial basal hypothalamus, *Brain Res.,* 405, 384, 1987.

37. Steinhilber, D., Brungs, M., Werz, O., Weisenberg, I., Danielsson, C., Kahlen, J., Nayeri, S., Schrader, M., and Carlberg, C., The nuclear receptor for melatonin represses 5-lipooxygenase gene expression in human B lymphocytes, *J. Biological Chem.,* 270, 7037, 1995.

38. Maurizi, C.P., The loss of intraventricular fluid melatonin can explain the neuropathology of Alzheimer's disease, *Med. Hypotheses,* 49, 153, 1997.

39. Blass, J.P., Cerebral metabolic impairments, in Khachaturian, Z.S. and Rabebaugh, T.S., Eds., *Alzheimer's Disease. Cause(s), Diagnosis, Treatment and Care,* CRC Press, Boca Raton, FL, 1996, 187.

40. Halliwell, B., Oxidants and the central nervous system: some fundamental questions, *Acta Neurol. Scand.,* 126, 23, 1989.

41. Zhou, Y., Richardson, J.S., Mombourquette, M.J., and Weil, J.A., Free radical formation in autopsy samples of Alzheimer and control cortex, *Neurosci. Lett.,* 1995, 89, 1995.

42. Halliwell, B., Reactive oxygen species and the central nervous system, *J. Neurochem.,* 59, 1609, 1992.

43. Smith, C.D., Carney, J.M., Tatsumo, T., Stadtman, E.R., Floyd, R.A., and Markesbery, W.R., Protein oxidation in aging brain, *Ann. N.Y. Acad. Sci.,* 663, 110, 1992.

44. Smith, M.A., Richey, P.I., Taneda, S., Kurry, R.K., Sayre, L.M., Monnier, V.M., and Perry, G., Advanced Maillard reaction end products, free radicals, and protein oxidation in Alzheimer's disease, *Ann. N.Y. Acad. Sci.,* 738, 447, 1994.

45. Mecocci, P., MacGarvey, U., and Beal, M.F., Oxidative damage to mitochondrial DNA is increased in Alzheimer's disease, *Ann. Neurol.,* 36, 747, 1994.

46. Pappolla, M.A., Omar, R.A., Kim, K.S., and Robakis, N.K., Immunohistochemical evidence of antioxidant stress in Alzheimer's disease, *Am. J. Pathol.,* 140, 621, 1992.

47. Parker, W.D., Parks, J., Filley, C.M., and Kleinschmidt-DeMasters, B.K., Electron transport chain defects in Alzheimer's disease brain, *Neurology,* 44, 1090, 1994.

48. Corral-Debrinski, M., Horton, T., Lott, M.T., Shoffner, J.M., McKee, A.C., Beal, M.F., Graham, B.H., and Wallace, D.C., Marked changes in mitochondrial DNA deletion levels in Alzheimer brain, *Genomics,* 23, 471, 1994.

49. Good, P.F., Werner, P., Hsu, A., Onanow, C.W., and Perl, D.P., Evidence for neuronal oxidative damage in Alzheimer's disease, *Am. J. Pathol.,* 149, 21, 1996.

50. Blass, J.P., Baker, A.C., and Black, R.S., Induction of Alzheimer antigens by an uncoupler of oxidative phosphorylation, *Arch. Neurol.,* 47, 864, 1990.

51. Thompson, C.D., Apoptosis in the pathogenesis and treatment of disease, *Science,* 267, 1456, 1995.

52. Smale, G., Nichols, N.R., Brady, E.R., Finch, C.E., and Horton, W.E., Evidence for apoptotic cell death in Alzheimer's disease, *Exp. Neurol.,* 133, 225, 1995.

53.   Gagnoli, C.M., Atabay, C., Kharlamova, E., and Manev, H., Melatonin protects neurons from singlet oxygen-induced apoptosis, *J. Pineal Res.,* 18, 222, 1995.

54.   Cagnacci, A., Elliott, J.A., and Yen, S.S.C., Melatonin: a major regulator of circadian rhythm of core temperature in humans, *J. Clin. Endocrinol. Metab.,* 75, 447, 1992.

55.   Deacon, S. and Arendt, J., Melatonin-induced temperature suppression and its acute phase-shifting effects correlate in dose-dependent manner in humans, *Brain Res.,* 668, 77, 1995.

56.   Souetre, E., Salvati, E., Belugou, J. L., Krebs, B., and Darcourt, G., 5-methoxypsoralen as a specific stimulating agent of melatonin secretion in humans, *J. Clin. Endocrinol. Metab.,* 71, 670, 1990.

57.   Souetre, E., Salvati, E., Krebs, B., Belugou, J., and Darcourt, G., Abnormal response to 5-methoxypsoralen in dementia, *Am J. Psychiatry,* 146, 1037, 1989.

58.   Brzezinski, A., Melatonin in humans, *New Engl. J. Med.,* 336, 186, 1997.

INDEX

Winter-like responses, 116
Women runners, 86

X

Xenopus
    embryos, 9
    melanophores, 5